THE
COMPLETE
BODY MASSAGE
COURSE

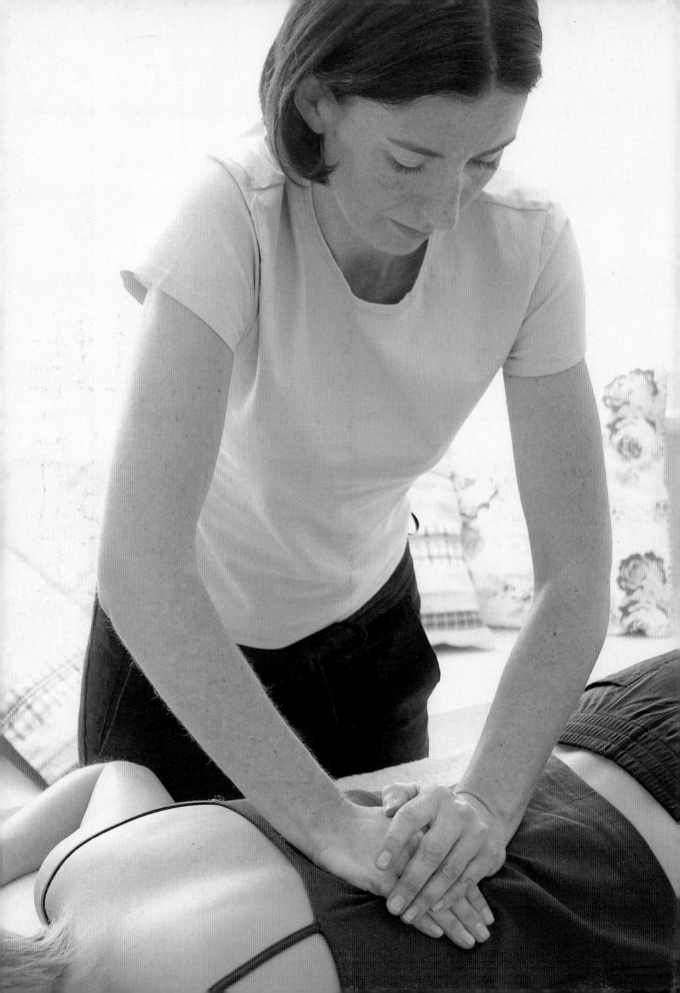

THE COMPLETE BODY MASSAGE COURSE

First published in Great Britain in 2006 by
Collins & Brown
The Chrysalis Building
Bramley Road
London W10 6SP

1 3 5 7 9 8 6 4 2

British Library Cataloguing-in-Publication Data:
A catalogue record for this book is available from the
British Library.

ISBN 1 84340 319 6

Commissioning Editor: Victoria Alers-Hankey
Editor: Jane Ellis
Design: Austin Taylor
Photographs: Guy Hearn
page 24: Michael Wicks

Reproduction by Anorax Imaging Limited
Printed and bound by Wing King Tong Co Limited, China

Acknowledgments
My thanks and appreciation to my family for their huge
encouragement and generosity. To my clients for their
loyalty and enthusiasm in my work. To Victoria Alers-
Hankey for making this book possible. And finally, my
special thanks to Stephen for his support and hands.

CONTENTS

HISTORY OF MASSAGE

Massage – the manipulation of the body's soft tissues –
is one of the oldest techniques of healing and seems to have been in
use since the days of early mankind. The word "massage" originates from several
different languages, including Latin, Greek and Arabic. In many cultures, and even for
many animals, massage manifests as a basic instinctive reaction – providing
reassurance and comfort in response to pain, easing stress or muscular tension and
speeding healing. In the East, ancient Chinese, Indian and Japanese manuscripts
refer to the use of massage to prevent and cure disease and to heal injury. In the
West, we have the words of the physician Hippocrates from the fifth century BC:
"rubbing can bind a joint that is too loose and loosen a joint that is too tight... can
make flesh or cause parts to waste; hard rubbing binds, soft rubbing loosens."
More recently, a Swedish fencing master named Per Henrik Ling (1776–1839)
developed a system of techniques upon which modern massage is largely based.
Since the start of the twentieth century massage has become increasingly popular
as people search for alternative ways of dealing with stress and health issues. This
has resulted in more emphasis being placed on the pleasurable and relaxing
potential of massage, as well as its physical benefits.

There are many different types of massage and bodywork, all of which involve the
application of various techniques to stimulate the muscular structure and soft
tissues of the body.

Massage can be broken into broadly Western and Eastern categories. Western
methods, for example, wwedish massage, sports massage and deep tissue massage,
work mainly on the external physical body and involve the application of soft tissue
manipulation through five basic techniques. Eastern methods, including Shiatsu,
acupressure, Thai massage and Tui Na, are used to assess and restore the vital flow
of energy through "meridians" or energy channels.

In addition to these, there are a range of other massage-related therapies such as
energy-based treatments like Polarity therapy and Reiki, which work on the body's
energy field and involve either the application of pressure or the holding of hands on

or above the body. Structural re-alignment methods such as the Alexander Technique place an emphasis on the structure and movement of the body in relationship to gravity and involve the correction of inappropriate patterns of posture and movement.

The benefits of massage are many and deep: it can help relieve and prevent chronic pain, lowered vitality and recurring infections; it can help conditions such as migraines, digestive disorders, hypertension and high blood pressure; it can be used to improve postural alignment and sports performance; and it promotes a sense of equilibrium. In the modern world where we suffer increasingly from emotional, mental and physical stresses, massage is one of the best ways to retrieve a sense of balance and reduce our feelings of anxiety.

The treatment time of a massage will vary between different methods but is usually between 30 and 90 minutes. Massage can be carried out either with or without lubricants and the person being treated may be fully clothed, partly clothed or naked, according to the method employed.

Over the years massage teachers and therapists will master their own distinct and favoured methods of practice; many will also train in various methods and may combine techniques to produce a treatment to suit the individual or location. On-site massage, for example, combines techniques that are tailored for the ease and convenience of the work place.

It must be remembered that massage cannot be learnt from simply reading about the theory. Whilst each technique in this book has been explained and illustrated with care, what follows is a basic introduction, not a complete teaching course. As you do more massage your confidence will gradually increase and your skills will develop. You will learn most by getting feedback from the people you massage. It is extremely important to be aware of all "contraindications" (symptoms that could be aggravated by massage), which are given on pages 10–11. If in any doubt, do not give a massage before consulting a doctor or a specific practitioner.

1

THE
BASICS

1. How to use this book

WHO IS IT DESIGNED FOR?

This book is a convenient and easy guide for anyone who is interested in the amazingly broad world of massage and for those who would like to explore the various techniques and treatments to practise on themselves, their family or friends at home. It is not aimed at professional practitioners, nor is it designed to give the kind of in-depth knowledge that most therapists acquire over years of practise. For each therapy in the book, there is a selection of step-by-step techniques – illustrated with photographs. You may wish to complete an entire sequence or simply practise a few of the steps to get you started.

WHAT IS IT DESIGNED FOR?

The book provides a comprehensive introduction to the best-known therapies, including their history, principles, basic practices and typical techniques. There is a directory of professional organizations to help you find a suitable practitioner or course, if you are interested in exploring a particular technique further or in training to become a bodywork therapist yourself.

2. Safety guidance and contraindications

BEFORE FOLLOWING ANY MASSAGE SEQUENCE, it is important that you understand the following safety guidelines by considering any possible contraindications. Contraindications are situations in which massage could aggravate a problem or jeopardize the health of the recipient. Properly used, massage is unlikely to cause any adverse reactions, but applying too much deep pressure or over-treating a particular area could, for example, cause inflammation to sensitive skin or muscle tissue. There are times when massage should be avoided altogether, or at least significantly modified. You should never try to diagnose a health problem for yourself or anyone else. Remember, if in doubt, a qualified medical practitioner should always be consulted.

Total contraindications, i.e. massage should not be given to:

◆ A pregnant woman during the first three months and massage involving the use of aromatherapy products should not be given to a mother who is breastfeeding, unless supervized by a professional practitioner.

◆ Anyone who is under the influence of alcohol or recreational drugs.

◆ Sufferers of thrombosis (massage could dislodge a blood clot, resulting in fatal consequences) or those who have cancer (unless they have permission from their doctor).

Localized contraindications, i.e. massage should avoid certain areas:

◆ Open wounds, broken bones, bruises, joint dislocation or soft tissue ruptures.

◆ Areas of major inflammation where there is heat, redness or burns.

◆ Areas of swelling caused by arthritis, gout, gastritis, appendicitis, neuritis or bursitis.

◆ Areas of infections: viral (herpes, warts); bacterial (acne, boils and skin conditions) or fungal (athlete's foot).

◆ Any undiagnosed lumps or bumps or areas of pain.

◆ Varicose veins – in advanced cases massage should be avoided; in minor cases very light pressure may be applied, but deep pressure will cause further damage to the vein.

People will often forget to tell you about accidents, injuries or ailments, so it is always a good idea to run through the following questions with the person you are going to massage. This will establish if there are any conditions that they have forgotten to tell you about and that all possible contraindications have been properly considered.

◆ Are they taking any medication? If so, what is it for? For example, do they have high or low blood pressure? Be aware that someone with blood pressure problems may feel dizzy when they move.

◆ Have they had any recent accidents? Examples include whiplash or broken bones. Establish that a doctor has examined them.

◆ Are they asthmatic? Make sure you know where they keep their inhaler.

◆ Have they eaten recently? It's wise for both the giver and the receiver to avoid big meals immediately before or after a massage.

◆ If the recipient is a woman, is she pregnant? Note the contraindications given above for pregnancy.

If the person you are massaging has any symptoms that persist or worsen, stop the treatment immediately and advise them to consult a doctor.

3.Setting up the work space

MASSAGE CAN BE PRACTISED ALMOST ANYWHERE, but in order to give the maximum benefit, it is important to create a warm, tranquil environment where your recipient will feel comfortable. Many people enjoy listening to music while having a massage, but do check with them first.

Massage should be carried out on a firm padded surface. This can be a specifically designed massage couch or chair, but a suitable ordinary table or chair, or even the floor (if properly padded) can all be utilized. Each technique in the Massage Therapies section will state the most appropriate surface.

If you are using a massage couch or an ordinary table, it should be at a height between the middle and top of your thigh. You need to be able to lean into the table with your body weight without twisting or slouching and your upper back should be straight at all times, to avoid putting it under undue strain.

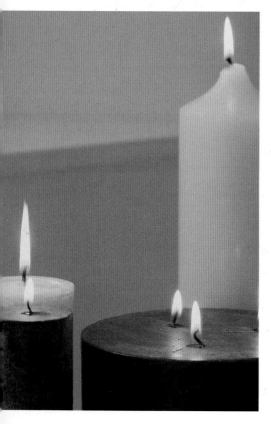

It is important to make sure your that table is sufficiently strong to bear the weight of the person you intend to massage, taking into account the pressure you may exert during the treatment. If you are massaging on the floor or a futon, pad it with plenty of towels and/or blankets so it is comfortable for both you and the recipient.

Placing a pillow under the recipient's knees when they are lying face up – and under their ankles when they are lying face down – will help to relax both their lower back and stomach. If you are using a chair and do not have one specifically designed for massage, ask the recipient to sit astride an ordinary dining chair and pad the back with a cushion so that they can comfortably lean forward.

If you are giving an unclothed massage, keep the recipient covered at all times with a towel, sheet or blanket; only the area you are massaging should be exposed. Try to avoid working under harsh ceiling lights. Make sure your nails are short, your hands are clean and any jewellery is removed.

Relax when you are massaging and allow your fingers to seek out tight or knotted areas. With regular practise, your sensitivity and confidence will grow. Try to keep one of your hands in contact with the recipient's body at all times and always invite feedback – your techniques should never make someone feel uncomfortable or cause pain. When you have finished the session, let the person you've massaged rest for a few minutes before they try to get up or move. Encourage them to drink plenty of water, as this will help to flush out toxins and rehydrate the body.

4.Massage oils and lubricants

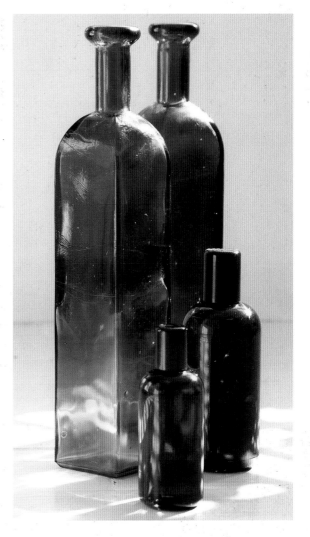

OILS, LOTIONS AND POWDERS ARE USED to help the hands glide easily over the skin. Lubricants are not used for pressure point massage or clothed massage. Each therapy in Part 2 will give advice on which lubricant is the best for that technique. (Aromatherapy oils are covered in more detail on pages 22–23).

Vegetable oils, such as grapeseed, almond and avocado are some of the most frequently used oils because the skin easily absorbs them. They are readily available in most health stores and larger supermarkets. It can be difficult at first to judge how much oil you need. Start by pouring a little oil into the palm of one hand, rub your hands together to warm the oil and then apply the hands to the body. Continue adding small amounts of oil as necessary throughout the massage. Using too much oil can prevent good control of the hands, while too little oil may irritate the skin by pulling the hairs.

If you are going to give a reflexology treatment, talcum powder is the most popular medium and is used to avoid skin traction.

5. Anatomy basics

THE STRUCTURE OF THE BODY principally consists of the skeleton and the muscles, some of which are "voluntary" (under our conscious control), such as the muscles of the legs and arms, which we can move at will. Other muscles are "involuntary" (not under our conscious control), for example, the muscles of the heart.

The skeleton is made up of 206 bones, which protect our internal organs and provide the framework for movement. Bones are linked to joints by ligaments (flexible bands of fibrous connective tissue).

Skeletal muscles are composed of muscle and nerve fibres bound together by connective tissue. They are attached to bone by a tendon at an origin (an attachment to a bone which does not move) and an insertion (an attachment to a bone which does move).

Muscles work in pairs: as one contracts, the other relaxes; the contracted muscle provides movement whilst the relaxed muscle provides stability and balance. Muscles need oxygen and glucose in order to provide movement and expel waste products, such as lactic acid, which are produced during vigorous or prolonged exercise. Stiff muscles are often a sign that the body has not expelled these waste products.

The skin is a regenerating organ and is the largest of the body. It is made up of an outer layer, the "epidermis", which largely contains skin cells and has no nerve endings. The underlying layer of connective tissue, the "dermis" contains blood, lymph and nerve vessels, as well as sweat glands and hair follicles. The skin regulates the body's temperature and protects it from infection. Skin is strengthened by the production of collagen and elastic fibres. If these fibres harden through stress, diet or injury, the molecules that make up the connective tissue bind together, making the skin less flexible.

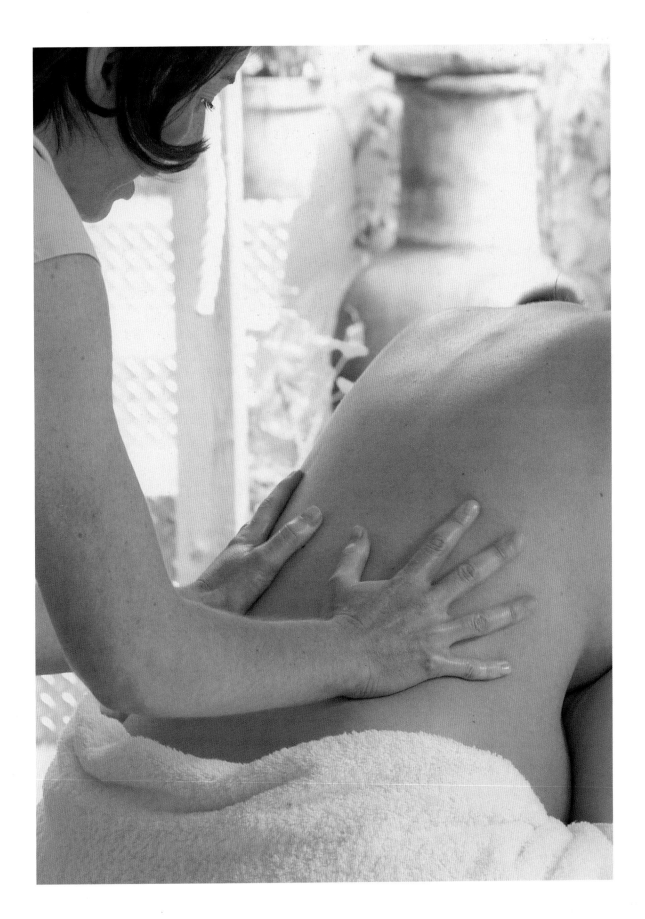

6.Massage techniques

Most massage therapies use a combination of the techniques described below. The application of these techniques varies according to the type of therapy. Most of the techniques can be used either in a brisk, invigorating way or slowly and gently, depending on the effect you are trying to achieve.

EFFLEURAGE (STROKING)

Effleurage is a stroking technique that forms the basis of all massages where oil is used. It is generally used to start and end a treatment and to link different techniques within the treatment. It allows you to apply the oil and warm the muscles and identifies areas of tension, while the recipient gets used to your touch. Effleurage boosts the circulation, clears the lymphatic system, maintains relaxation and aids in the elimination of toxins. Depending on the speed of the strokes, this technique can be either calming or invigorating.

Effleurage should be a fluid movement with both hands, either alongside each other or alternately with fingers and thumbs together or apart. You should try to cover the whole area being massaged and mould your hands into the contours of the body to apply long, sweeping movements both lengthways and across the body. The strokes are repeated so that the muscles become warmed and relaxed. Once you have established a rhythm, you may gradually increase the pressure. Ensure that all your strokes are directed towards the heart when treating the limbs; this will help the return of blood to the heart and improve lymph drainage.

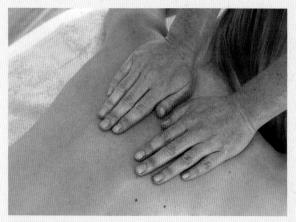 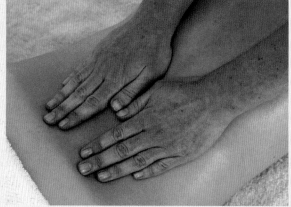

Initial touch Effleurage with both hands up and down the back, either side of the spine.

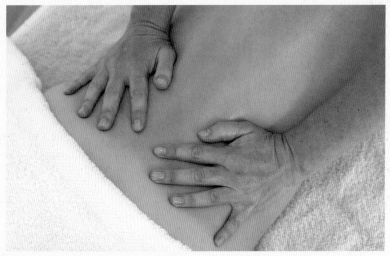

Effleurage with the fingers together or fanned.

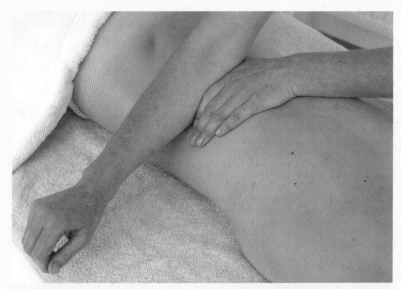

Forearm effleurage Place your elbow between the web of your thumb and forefinger and guide your forearm up or down the back, on either side of the spine.

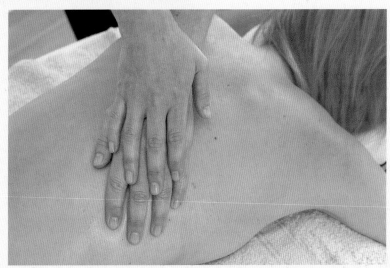

Transverse effleurage With hands on top of each other to increase the pressure, pull up and through the ribs.

PETRISSAGE (KNEADING/PALMING)

The technique for petrissage is similar to kneading bread; it uses the hands and fingers to break down tension. Particular areas or muscles are manipulated and compressed as both your hands work rhythmically. Start by slowly grasping the flesh with your hands; lift it, pulling slightly away from the bone, and then release. Immediately repeat the movement with the other hand, with the hands sliding the flesh towards each other. Continue to lift and release with alternate hands, ensuring your movements are smooth and you are not pinching the skin. As this technique can be quite tricky to master, work slowly to start with and gradually move around the area you want to treat.

Petrissage is used on large, pliable muscles such as shoulders, thighs and hips and can be applied in varying pressures. Don't use this technique on delicate or bony areas. It is an invigorating movement that breaks down tension and stiffness in both superficial and deep muscles, depending on the pressure applied. Petrissage is usually repeated throughout a massage in several different areas of the body; it is preceded and followed by effleurage to warm the muscles first and to clear the area of toxins afterwards. It helps to stretch muscles and boost circulation – a process that speeds the elimination of waste products such as lactic acid.

Grasp, squeeze and release the muscles, as if you were kneading dough.

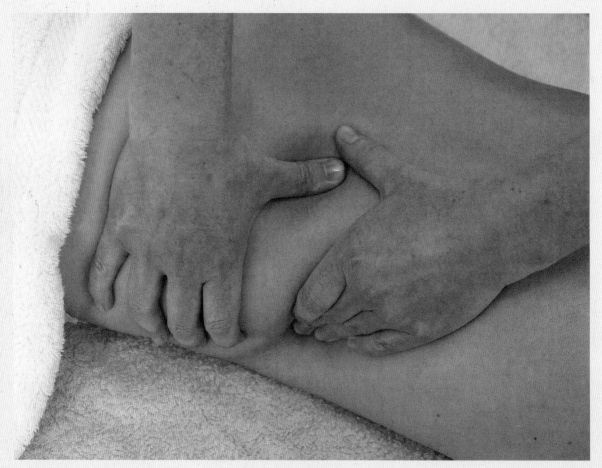

FRICTION

Friction is a deep, rubbing technique that is applied to localized areas of knottiness or scar tissue. It is very good for releasing tension in muscles and loosening tightness. Start by placing the pads of your thumbs or your fingertips on the area concerned and apply a firm pressure, using your bodyweight to help you. Slowly trace small circles in a rubbing movement. Work a small area, trying to break down the tension before moving on. You could try moving your thumbs/fingers up and down or just apply static pressure.

Great sensitivity is needed when using friction; it is important to get feedback from your recipient – you should never go in too deep, work too fast or spend too long on an area, as pain and bruising may be caused. Friction must always be followed by effleurage to clear the area of toxins and relax the muscles. As well as breaking down areas of scar tissue and tension, friction helps to warm up an area, boosts circulation and enhances the flexibility of the muscles.

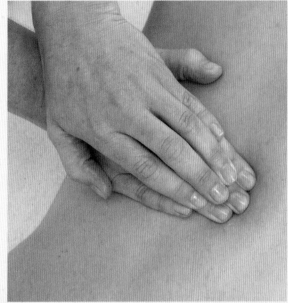

Finger friction With the pads of your fingers, placing one hand on top of the other will help to guide your fingers and increase pressure.

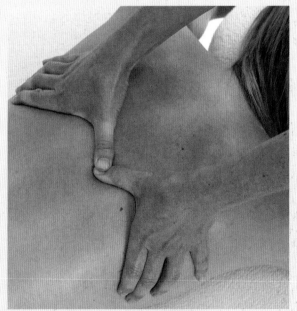

Thumb friction Using only your thumbs, press the pads of your thumbs into the muscles and slowly friction in circular or transverse movements.

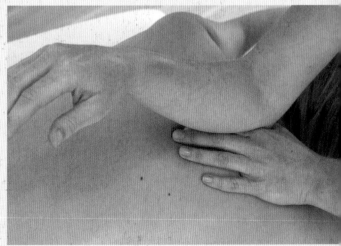

Elbow friction Using controlled pressure with the elbow, place your elbow between the web of your thumb and forefinger and friction. Take great care not to apply too much pressure or friction over bone.

TAPOTEMENT, HACKING AND CUPPING (PERCUSSION)

Percussion techniques are brisk, energizing movements. You use your hands to repeatedly strike the body lightly and rapidly.

◆ **Tapotement** is a very gentle form of percussion, using only the fingertips. It is good for using on the face. With relaxed wrists, apply quick, light taps with your fingers, keeping the movements delicate.

◆ **Hacking or chopping** is the classic Swedish massage technique. With your palms facing each other and fingers slightly open, quickly strike the body with alternate hands, keeping the movements relaxed and bouncy. Gradually build into a more invigorating pace.

◆ **Cupping** is a similar technique used with your hands slightly rounded to form the shape of cups. It is particularly efficient as it creates a vacuum on the skin as the hands move briskly off the body.

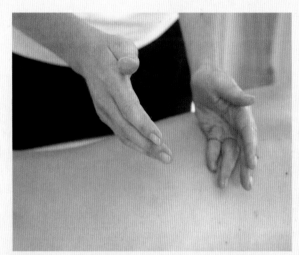

Percussion boosts circulation, stimulates the muscle tissues and is invigorating at the end of a massage, when it is most frequently used. As with all percussion techniques, be careful not to slap the skin.

Hacking With relaxed fingers and wrists, strike the body with the outer edges of your hands. This technique can be done with your hands working alternately or with them held together in a praying position. Your wrists must be loose so that the technique never becomes too hard.

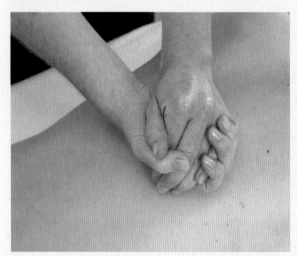

Cupping Cup your hands together to form a shallow pocket of air and strike the skin in quick successive movements. Ensure that you do not slap the skin.

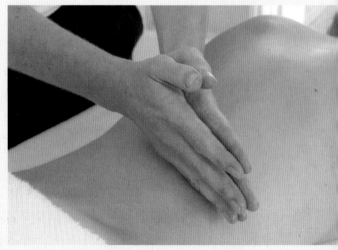

Hands together Outside border striking the skin alternately – fingers and wrists loose and relaxed.

SQUEEZING

Squeezing is used in both clothed and unclothed massage and is most frequently used to treat the limbs. Use both hands together interlocked to squeeze the muscle between your fingers and thumb, or with the flat of your fingers and palm. Two muscles can be squeezed in opposite directions, for example, the bicep and tricep muscles of the arm; or it can be used to treat one muscle, for example, the pulling up and squeezing of the calf muscle. Squeezing is used to stimulate the circulation and relax the muscles.

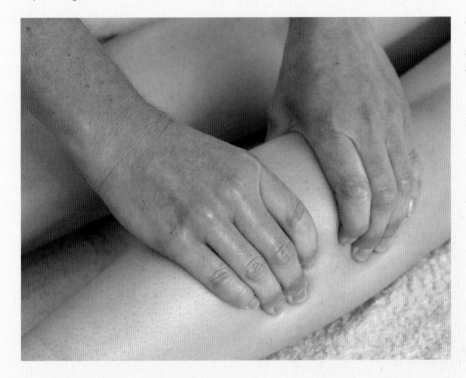

Squeeze the calf between your fingers and thumbs or fingers and palms.

PALMING

Palming is a relaxing technique that is used to warm, stretch and stimulate the muscles. It is the most common technique used for massage treatments that are given with the recipient clothed. Using your body weight, pressure is applied with the palms of your hands to create stationary pressure and stretch the muscles. Palming can be applied simultaneously, alternately, with one hand on top of the other to apply a wavelike deeper action or in circular rotations to knead the muscle.

PLUCKING

Plucking is a deep technique that is used in Tui Na to relax a muscle and ease tension. Use the pad of your thumb to apply deep pressure across a muscle. Place the heel of your opposite hand on top of the thumb to guide and push the thumb backward and forward across the muscle in a kneading action.

7.Aromatherapy basics

Essential oils may be used in the bath in hot or cold compresses, mixed into creams, lotions, aromatic waters and carrier oils, or in a diffuser to fill a room with scent.

BACKGROUND

Aromatherapy is the use of aromatic plant essences (known as essential oils) to maintain and promote health and balance in the body. Herbs and essential oils have been used for thousands of years – for healing, embalming, in religious ceremonies and as perfume. The antiseptic power of certain essences had been recognized by the Middle Ages, but it was the chemist and perfume manufacturer Rene Maurice Gattefosse who coined the word "aromatherapy" in the 1920s. After sustaining a severe burn to his hand, he applied lavender oil to it and found that it healed without leaving a scar. He subsequently studied and began to formulate the medicinal benefits of oils from various plants and applied through massage, as an additive in the bath or as an inhalation. Aromatherapy began to be used as a treatment during the 1950s.

Aromatherapy oils are extracted from herbs, flowers, grasses, woods and roots with unique characteristics and benefits. The oils enter and leave the human body easily without leaving toxins. They have many different properties: relaxing, invigorating, antibacterial, anti-inflammatory or antiseptic. Lavender, for example, is antiseptic and calming and is beneficial for insomnia, headaches, cuts and grazes. It is one of the few oils (tea tree is another) that can be used undiluted directly on the skin to treat burns, stings and cuts. Some oils, including lemon and peppermint, are known as "adaptogens". They create equilibrium in the body and can therefore be listed as both a relaxant and a stimulant.

Essential oils may be used in the bath, in hot or cold compresses, mixed into creams, lotions, aromatic waters and carrier oils, or in a diffuser to fill a room with scent. All of these methods make aromatherapy an ideal first-aid treatment and a great complement to massage. Nevertheless, essential oils can have very powerful effects, which vary with the individual. If you wish to use aromatherapy, exercise due caution and care. The quality and cost of essential oils also varies greatly and you should try to use the purest highest-quality oil possible.

MASSAGING

An aromatherapy massage is principally the same as a traditional Swedish massage, but with the use of essential oils. The massage encourages the essential oil to be absorbed into the body via the skin.

BLENDING

Essential oils must be diluted with a carrier or base oil unless otherwise specified. The best base oils are cold pressed vegetable oils, such as sweet almond, grape seed or sunflower. A blend will consist of between 15 and 30 drops of essential oil mixed with 50 ml/2.5 fl oz of carrier oil (weaker dilutions should be used for sensitive skin). The oils can often complement and enhance each other's actions and up to four different oils may be used in a blend. All oils are categorized into "notes" – a measure of their evaporation speed. A top note will make an initial impact and then evaporate quickly; a middle note lasts longer and a base note has the most staying power. For a fragrance to last the length of a massage, the blend should contain oils with top, middle and base notes. Keep the blended mixture in a dark glass bottle, out of direct sunlight.

BATHING

Typically, six to eight drops of neat essential oils or one to two teaspoons of a blend should be added to a bath when it has been run.

INHALATION

Inhalation will occur naturally when bathing or massaging with essential oils. Other methods of inhalation are to add one to six drops of essential oil to a diffuser, a dish of water or a cotton wool ball placed over a radiator. The oils can also be simply dropped on a tissue and breathed in.

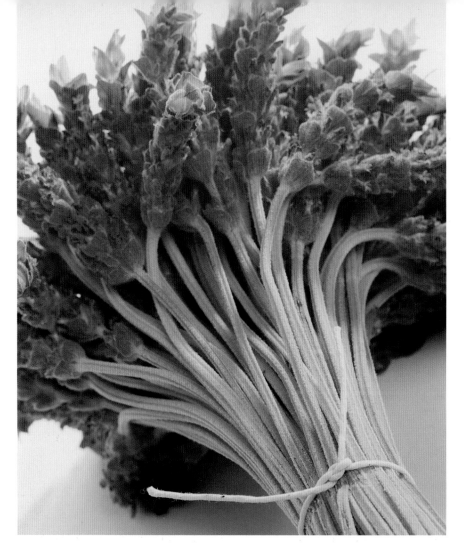

SOME COMMON ESSENTIAL OILS

◆ **LAVENDER (middle note):**
Antibiotic, antiseptic, anti-depressant, anti-inflammatory, analgesic, protects against infection, anti-spasmodic, balancing, relaxant, sedative and detoxifying. It is one of the most commonly used oils, effective for treating headaches, insomnia, anxiety and wounds. It can be used neat.

◆ **TEA TREE (top note):**
Analgesic, antiseptic, anti-inflammatory, antiviral, antibacterial and antifungal. It is used for treating infections, sunburn, acne, athlete's foot and toothache.

◆ **PEPPERMINT (middle note):**
Analgesic, anti-inflammatory, antiseptic, antiviral, antibacterial, hormonal, stimulant, digestive. It is used to treat indigestion, flatulence, flu, headaches, skin irritations, toothache and fatigue. It boosts the circulation and aids respiration. It should be used in low concentrations and not on children.

◈ ROMAN CHAMOMILE (middle note):

Analgesic, antibacterial, antiseptic, anti-inflammatory, calming, diuretic, relaxant and sedative. It treats teething problems, burns, asthma, eczema, hay fever, diarrhoea, sprains and strains, nausea, fever and psoriasis. It is the best oil for children.

◈ EUCALYPTUS (top note):

Antifungal, anti-inflammatory, antiseptic, antiviral, diuretic, analgesic and deodorizing. It is used to treat coughs, colds, cystitis, candida, diabetes, sunburn and as an insect repellent.

◈ GERANIUM (middle note):

Analgesic, antifungal, anti-infectious, anti-inflammatory, astringent, bactericidal, balancing, relaxant and stimulant. It is soothing, cooling, balances the emotions and is used to treat menopausal problems, diabetes, throat infections and as a nerve tonic and sedative.

◈ ROSEMARY (middle note):

Analgesic, antiseptic, antispasmodic, antibacterial, diuretic. It is a physical and mental stimulant, muscular relaxant and is used to treat fluid retention, headaches, coughs and flu.

◈ THYME (middle note):

Antiviral, antibiotic, antiseptic and diuretic. It should be used in moderation, never applied undiluted or on children. It is used to treat flu, warts, fatigue and acne and is very effective in a diffuser as an insect repellent.

◈ LEMON (top note):

Antiseptic, antibacterial, anti-inflammatory, antiviral, astringent, balancing, diuretic, relaxant, stimulant and digestive. Lemon is uplifting and calming and is used to treat insect bites and some fungal infections.

◈ CLOVE (middle note):

Antibacterial, antifungal, antiviral, antiseptic, analgesic and a stimulant. It helps to prevent the spread of infection, and is a well-known remedy for toothache, digestive disorders, asthma and sinusitis. It should never be used undiluted on skin.

8. Self-massage

Before starting a massage on a friend or partner, it is a great idea to practise on yourself first. A self-massage will not only increase your confidence and understanding of the different techniques, it will allow you to assess how various degrees of pressure feel and it will improve your finger sensitivity and rhythm. It is also a wonderful tool for the self-treatment of many minor ailments, injuries and stress.

TECHNIQUE

You will rarely apply the same pressure to yourself as you would to another person and it won't be possible to do some of the techniques effectively in a self-treatment. Make sure that your muscles are warm and relaxed before you start. You may have to move through different body positions to shorten and relax the area you want to massage, for example, bending your neck slightly to one side or positioning your elbow or foot on a table.

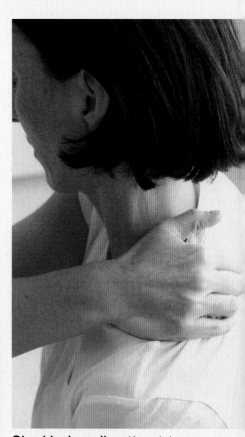

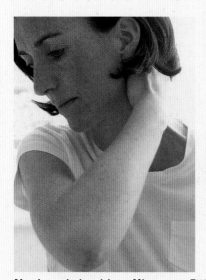 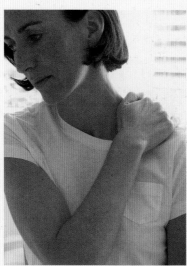

Neck and shoulder effleurage Either sitting or standing, cross one arm over your chest and use your fingers to stroke from the base of your skull down your neck and across to your shoulder. Repeat several times. Drop your head very slightly towards the opposite shoulder – this will stretch the neck and increase the impact of your massage. Repeat several times. Repeat on the other shoulder.

Shoulder kneading Knead down your neck and along the shoulder by squeezing the muscles between your palm and fingers. Repeat several times and follow with effleurage from step 1. Repeat on the other shoulder.

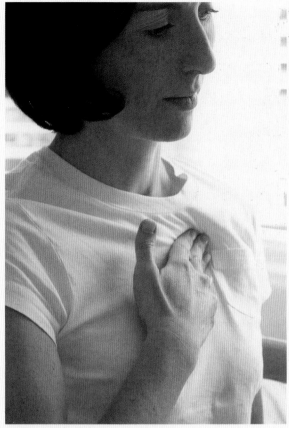

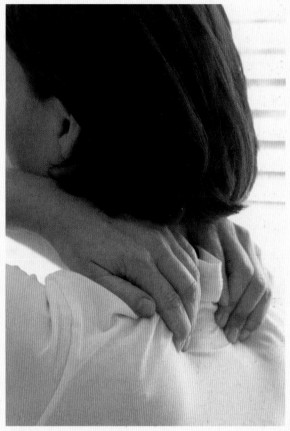

Chest massage Starting with your fingertips on your breastbone (sternum) and under your collarbone, effleurage out towards your shoulder. Pull your fingers back to your sternum. Repeat several times, your right hand massaging your left side. Swap hands to massage your right side. Massaging the chest helps to ease anxiety and induce relaxed breathing.

Shoulder kneading Place the heels of your hands at the base of your neck and drop your fingers down either side of your spine. Grasp the muscles with your fingertips, pull up and squeeze between your palms and fingers. Continue squeezing out towards the shoulders.

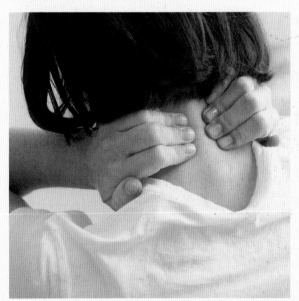

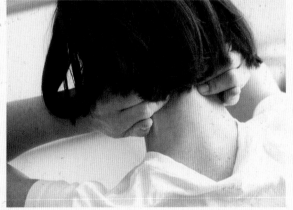

Neck kneading Wrap your fingers around the back of your neck. Pull the muscles away from spine and squeeze them between your palms and your fingers. Squeeze down the neck from the base of the skull to the base of the neck. Repeat several times.

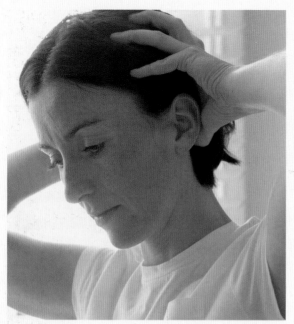

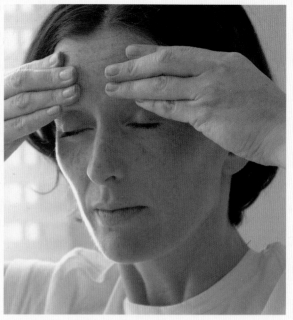

Friction around the base of the skull Place the pads of your thumbs directly under the base of the skull. With both hands in unison, apply small circular frictions up under the skull. Continue movements around to the ears.

Forehead massage Place your fingers in the centre of your forehead and draw your hands out to your temples. Massage your temples in slow circles with the pads of your fingers. Return your hands to the forehead and apply small circular frictions across to the temples. Repeat.

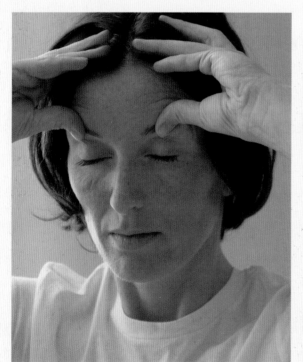

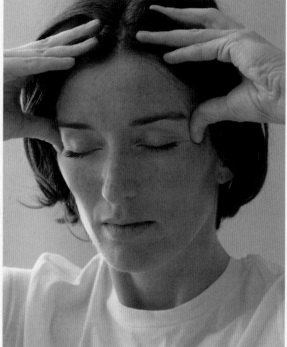

Eyebrow acupressure Press the pads of your thumbs into the bony rim of the eye sockets and hold for 10 seconds, move to the middle of the eyebrow (directly above the pupil) and hold for 10 seconds. Repeat at the end of the eyebrows and then circle the temples. Massaging around the eyes is wonderful for clearing eye tension.

Cheekbone acupressure

Place the pads of your fingers on the bridge of your nose and effleurage down to your cheek-bones. (Massaging down the nose is helpful in clearing congestion in the sinuses.) Now apply pressure to four points along your cheekbones with the pads of your thumbs. The first point is at the junction of the nose and the cheekbone, the second is directly below your pupil, the third point is in line with the end of the eyebrow and the fourth point is at the end of the cheekbone, just before the ear. Press up into each point and hold for 10 seconds. Repeat.

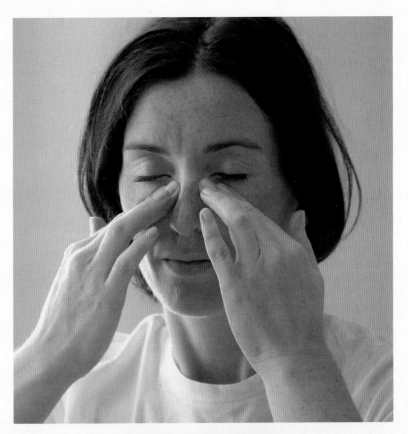

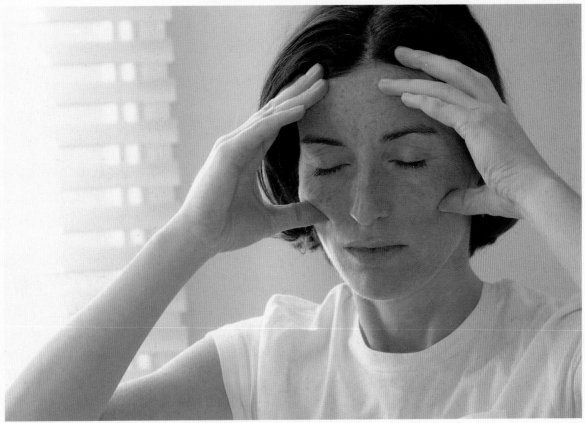

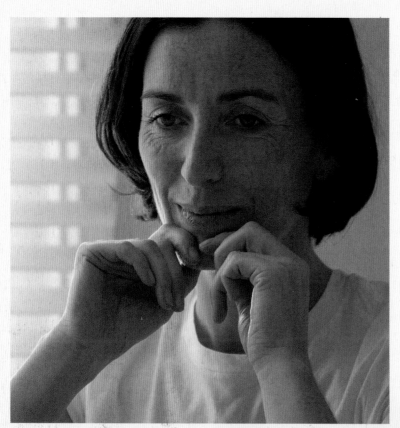

Jaw massage Place your index fingers in the centre of your chin and your thumbs under the jaw and massage in small circles around to your ears. Now pinch along the jaw line using your thumbs and the pad of your index fingers. Start in the centre of the chin and work out towards the ears. Hold each point for 10 seconds and repeat.

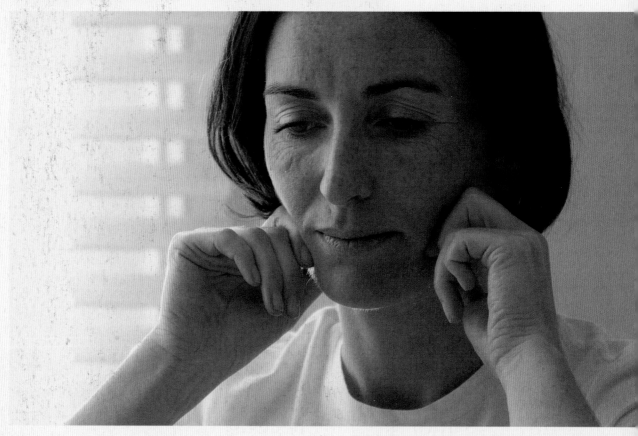

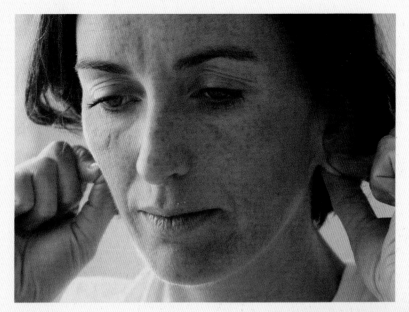

Head massage Squeeze your earlobes gently between your forefingers and thumbs. Repeat all over the ears and then massage up around behind the ears with the pads of your thumbs. To finish the treatment, comb your fingers up from your hairline to the top of your scalp and massage your scalp as if you were washing your hair.

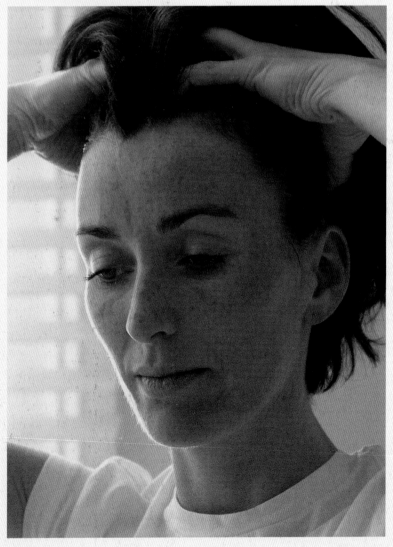

2

MASSAGE
THERAPIES

1.Swedish massage

Swedish massage is the manipulation of the superficial layers
of the muscles and soft tissues for therapeutic purposes.

BACKGROUND

Swedish massage was pioneered in the early nineteenth century by the
Swedish physiologist Per Henrik Ling. He found that a combination of
integrated movement and massage had a therapeutic effect on stiff joints. He
set up a clinic in Sweden, the Royal Central Institute of Gymnastics, where he
taught a series of gymnastic movements alongside massage. By the end of the
nineteenth century, Swedish massage had reached Britain where it became a
popular remedial treatment widely used by doctors and physiotherapists.
However, with the advent of physiotherapy machines, its use dwindled until
the 1970s when there was an increased awareness of the mind/body
connection and a renewed interest in using massage as a holistic therapy to
reduce emotional and physical stress. Today, Swedish massage is one of the
most commonly taught and well-known therapies and is the foundation for
many other forms of massage.

Swedish massage is the manipulation of the superficial layers of muscles
and soft tissues for therapeutic purposes. Its style is defined by the four
strokes: effleurage, petrissage, friction and percussion (see Massage
techniques, pages 16–21). It is designed to enhance the oxygen flow in the
blood and release toxins from the muscles, induce relaxation, enhance
flexibility and boost the circulation. Depending on the pressure applied, the
various techniques used either individually or in combination will affect the
skin, muscles, blood vessels, lymphatic system, the nervous system and some
of the body's internal organs. Fast movements are generally stimulating, while
slow ones have a calming and relaxing effect.

TECHNIQUE

A typical treatment with a professional masseur will last between an hour and
90 minutes. The therapist will take a thorough case history from every client
and will mentally note their posture, mobility and breathing. All the major
muscle groups will be massaged using oil or cream.

We have provided all the steps in the guided massage to do a full body
treatment, which will take approximately one hour. You may, however, choose

to concentrate on a specific area of the body or tailor the massage to fit in with the available time. You can do as many of the steps as you wish. You don't have to follow a set sequence or order, but starting on the back is usually pleasurable and instantly relaxing for the person you are massaging. When working on the arms and legs, it is important to direct your strokes toward the heart to follow the flow of blood back to the heart.

Try to make your massage sequence flow smoothly and remember to apply the techniques with sensitivity. Start with a light pressure, gradually increasing it to work deeper into areas of tension and knots – more time should be spent on problem areas. Never increase or decrease your massage pressure too suddenly and always ask the person you are massaging if the pressure you are applying is comfortable.

Have a good look at the person you are going to treat. What is their posture like? Are they slouching? Do the shoulders look hunched? Do they look twisted? Are they mobile or rigid? Is their breathing shallow or deep? By looking at the way a person moves and sits, you will start to learn to pinpoint areas of tension in the body.

Effleurage is the most commonly used technique in Swedish massage and will be returned to throughout a treatment.

The recipient should be undressed down to their underwear and (assuming you are going to start by massaging the back), lying face down on the massage couch or a suitably padded floor or table. Keep the recipient's body fully covered with a towel or sheet – remember that only the area being massaged should be exposed. Check that they are comfortable and warm.

Apply your chosen oil to the palm of your hands and rub them together vigorously to warm both them and the oil. Gently lay your hands on the person you are massaging and follow the first step. Once you have begun the massage, keep at least one of your hands in contact with the recipient's body until the end of the treatment. Encourage them to relax and breathe deeply, especially during deeper techniques when you should apply pressure on exhalation.

Before you start the guided massage, you should run through the list of contraindications on pages 10–11 with the person you are going to treat. If you are both confident there is no reason why the treatment should not be given, you can begin.

BENEFITS

Swedish massage is good for treating insomnia, general tension and headaches.

BASIC EFFLEURAGE

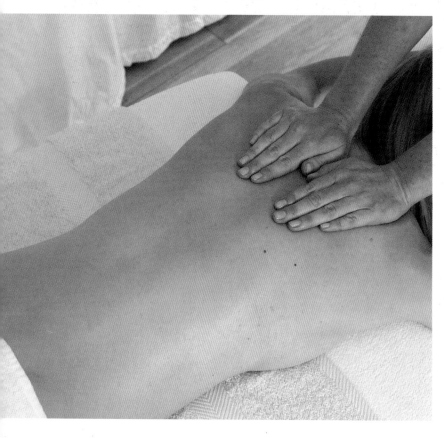

1 Before starting the back massage, stand at the side of your recipient and place one hand on the lower back and one on the upper back. Hold your hands in this position for up to 10 seconds, relaxing and focusing on your breathing. This will help both you and your recipient to relax.

When you're ready, pull the towel down as far as the top of the buttocks – a good way of securing it is to tuck it into the recipient's underwear. Start the massage by standing or kneeling at the recipient's head looking towards their feet. Apply oil to your hands, remembering to warm your hands and the oil by rubbing them vigorously together. With your fingertips and thumb together, place your hands on either side of the spine.

Lean your body weight into your hands and effleurage all the way down the back with a firm, even pressure. Do not apply pressure over the spine.

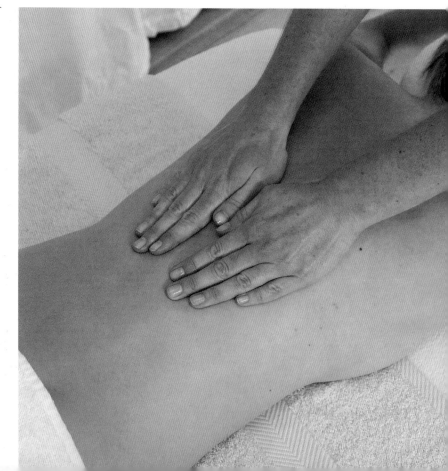

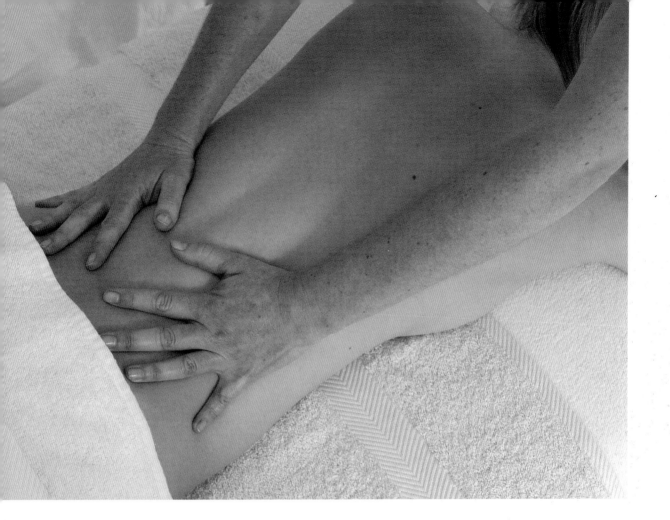

On reaching the lower back, fan your hands out and stroke down the sides of the body. Allow your hands to relax into the contours of the waist before pulling them back up towards the spine. Pull your hands up either side of the spine to return to step 1.

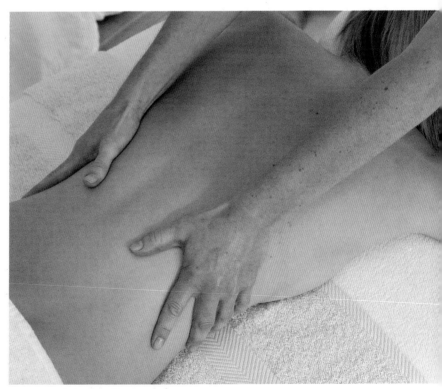

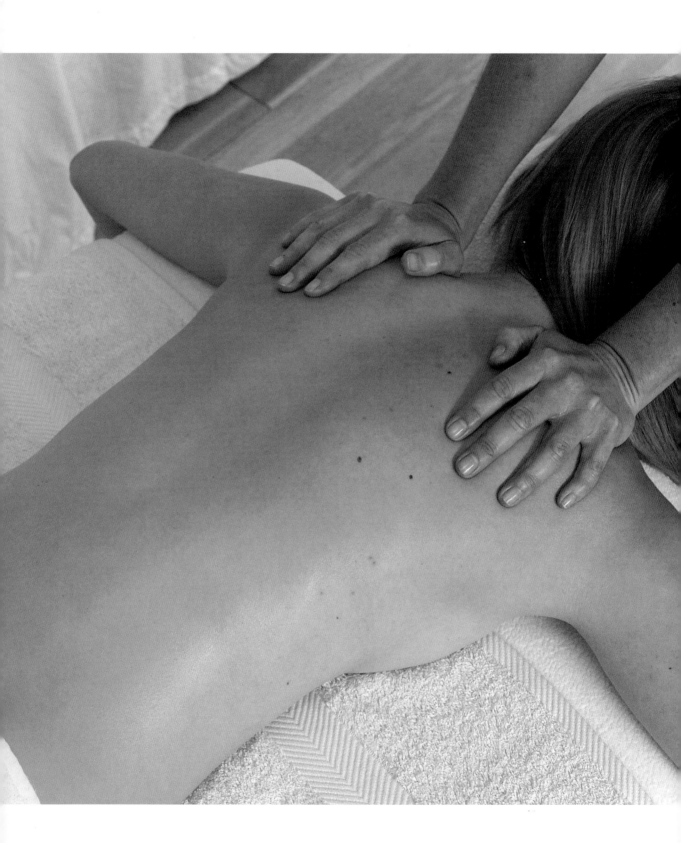

SHOULDER EFFLEURAGE

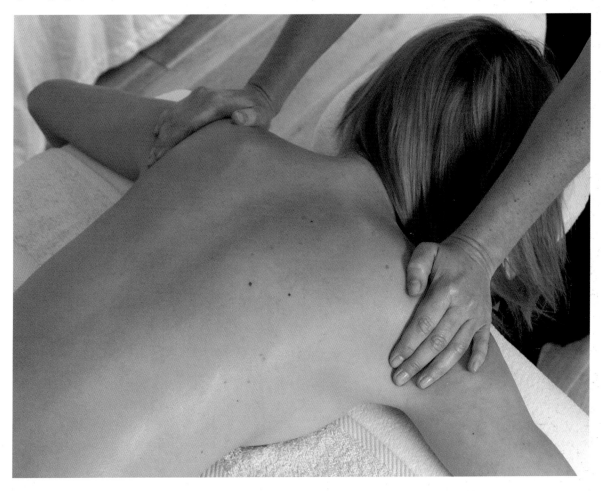

2 **Using the heels of your hands,** effleurage from the base of the neck across the shoulders and part way down the upper arm. Gently sweep your hands around and return to the starting position at the base of the neck.

Repeat steps 1–4 at least three times or until you feel that the back has been warmed up and the person you are treating is getting used to your touch and starting to relax. With effleurage, you can work with your fingers together or fanned, using both hands simultaneously, separately or alternately. You can apply long, light strokes or shorter, deep strokes; you can either relax or stimulate by using slow or fast movements. Remember when working on the back, to massage both up and down and transversally.

Effleurage is the most commonly used technique and it is used throughout a massage, so practise these moves on the back until you start to feel confident and build up a flowing rhythm.

SHOULDER KNEADING

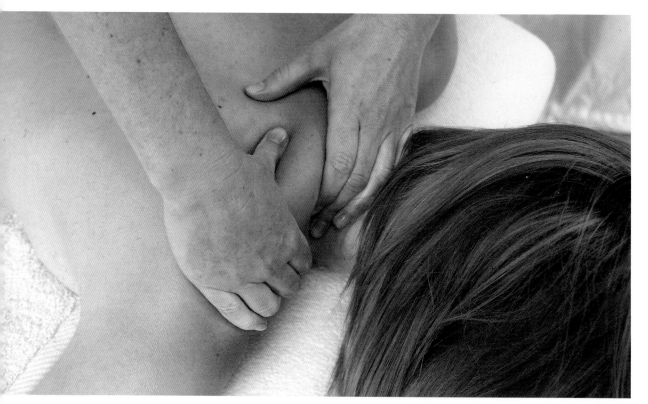

3 **Keeping one hand in contact** with the recipient's body, move to the left-hand side and stand facing the opposite shoulder. You are now going to do the petrissage technique. Knead the fleshy areas of the shoulder from the neck junction out. Repeat a couple of times and follow with effleurage.

Kneading helps to stimulate and relax areas of tension and can be used over any fleshy area of the back or buttocks, but remember to always follow kneading with effleurage.

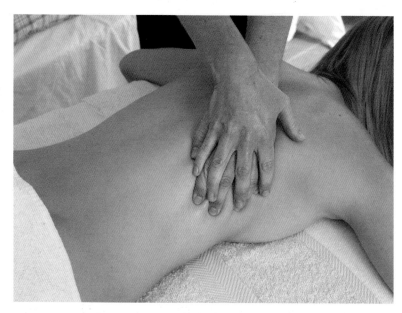

TRANSVERSE STROKE UP RIBS

4 **Place the pads of your fingers between the ribs** on the sides of the upper body and pull up and towards the spine. Placing one hand on top of the other will help you to guide your working hand and can be used to increase pressure. Repeat a couple of times.

SHOULDER BLADE EFFLEURAGE

5 **Slowly effleurage up and around** the fleshy border of the shoulder blade, continue up over the shoulder, down the upper arm and return to the starting position to repeat. Placing one hand on top of the other will help you to guide your working hand and can be used to increase the pressure applied.

Keep your hand in contact with the recipient's body and move to the opposite side to repeat steps 3, 4 and 5.

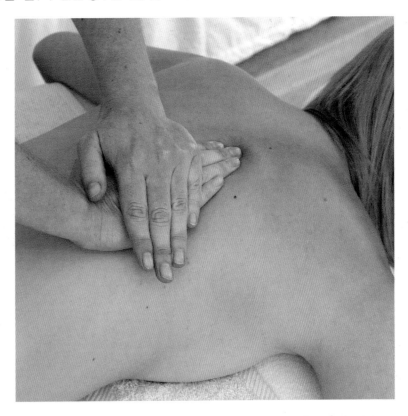

THUMB FRICTION

6 **Now return to the head of the recipient** and, facing their feet, place your thumbs on either side of their spine. Apply pressure using straight thumbs; this can be either stationary or in small circular, or back and forth movements. Start at the top of the spine and work down to the base. This is a good way of identifying areas of tension, which can be worked on for up to 30 seconds. Never overwork an area and always get feedback from the person you are treating. On reaching the base of the spine place your hands flat on the back and pull them up to the base of the neck. Then clear the area with a long effleurage stroke back down the spine.

Frictioning can be used around the shoulder blades, across the shoulders and around the base of the neck. Use caution when frictioning – with gradually increasing pressure – so that you don't accidentally hurt your recipient. Always follow with effleurage.

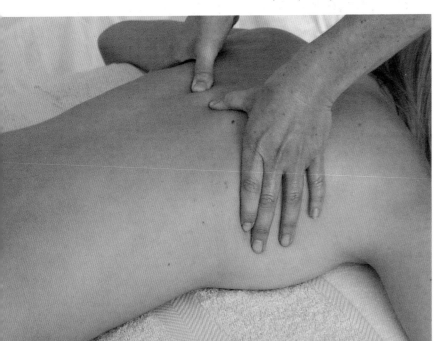

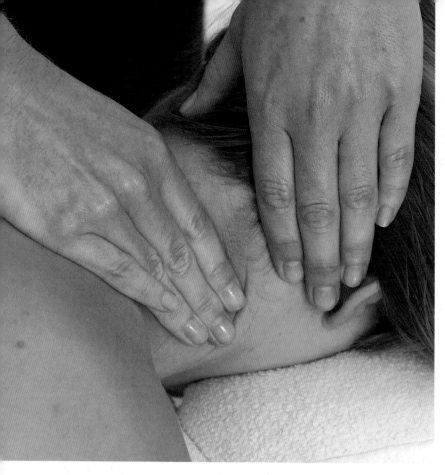

NECK EFFLEURAGE

7 **Standing on the left-hand side** of your recipient, effleurage up the neck to the base of the skull with the fingers and thumb of your right hand. The thumb of your hand will be facing you whilst your fingers will be on the right hand side of the neck. Rest your left hand on the recipient's head. Effleurage twice.

THUMB FRICTION AROUND THE BASE OF THE SKULL

8 **With your right thumb,** apply small circular frictions from the top of the spine up to the base of the skull and under the ears. Repeat several times. This area can be very tender, so take care not to work too deeply and remember never to apply pressure over bones. Massaging around the base of the skull and the neck is a wonderful way of easing tension and headaches. Keeping one hand in contact with the recipient, move around to the right-hand side and repeat steps 7 and 8.

Finish the back massage by repeating step 1. Pull up the towel to cover the back. Make sure the person you are treating feels warm enough before proceeding with the next steps. Remember that when you need more oil, apply it to your hands first.

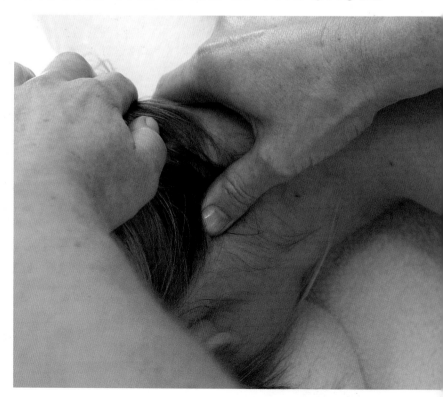

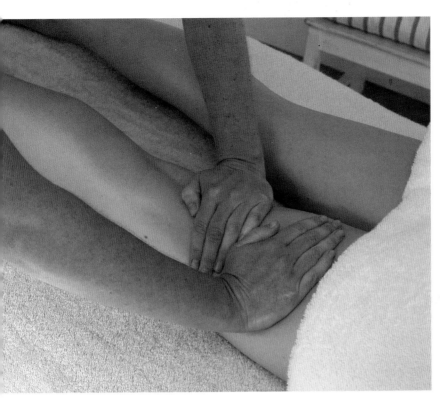

THIGH EFFLEURAGE

9 **Keeping one hand in contact** with the recipient's body, pull the towel up to the buttocks. Begin by applying effleurage from just above the back of the right knee up to the buttocks. Gently pull your hands back down either side of the thigh to return to the start. Repeat.

Make sure that you cover the outer, inner and mid-thigh, but keep clear of the groin area. Remember that you can work with fingers together or fanned, and with both hands working simultaneously, separately or alternately. When massaging the legs, apply the strokes upwards towards the heart and never apply pressure directly behind the knee.

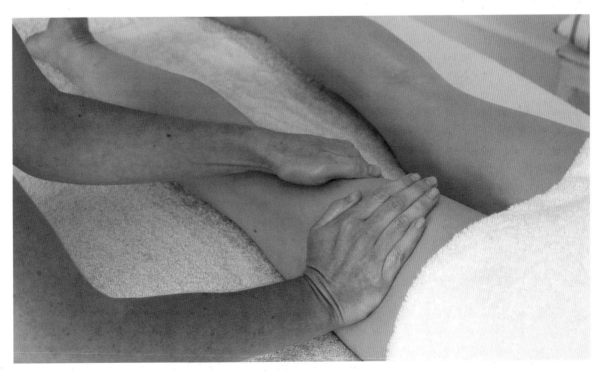

THIGH WRINGING

10 **With your hands on either side** of the thigh and fingers pointing away from you, pull one hand towards you as you push the other hand away. Repeat this crossing movement from the knee up to the buttocks.

THIGH KNEADING

11 **Knead up and down the thigh**, making sure you pay particular attention to the fleshy areas of the outer thigh. Your strokes should be slow and your hands should work rhythmically.

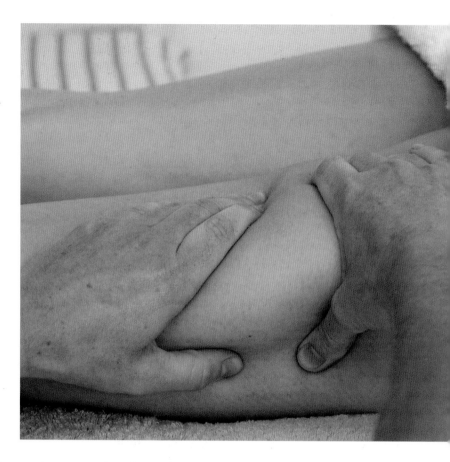

CALF MASSAGE

12 **Effleurage from the base of the calf muscle** to the buttocks. Repeat.

Now wrap your hands around the calf and, with your thumbs in the centre, slowly run them up the centre of the calf as if splitting the muscle. Repeat and follow with effleurage up to the buttocks.

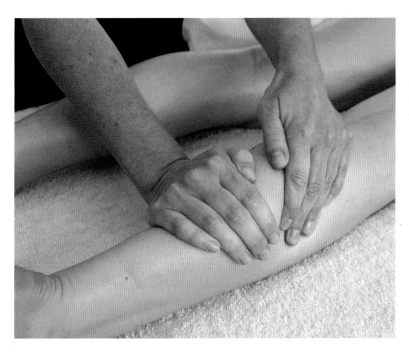

CALF WRING

13 **Wring the calf** using the same movements as you did for the thigh. As you push up with the heel of one hand, pull up with the fingers of the other and cross. Repeat to the knee.

VARIATION ON CALF EFFLEURAGE AND WRINGING

14 **Gently pick up the lower leg** and rest it on your inside shoulder. With your hands wrapped around the calf, effleurage it from the heel to the knee. Now wring the calf as in image 13. Elevating the lower leg aids the circulation of the blood and lymphatic systems.

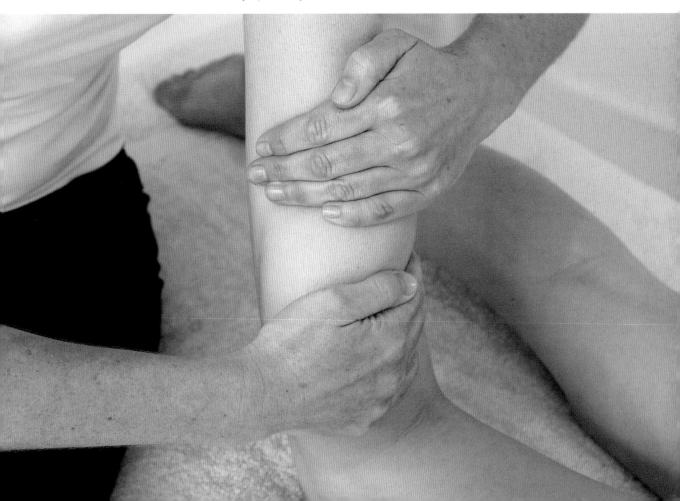

ELEVATED CALF FRICTION

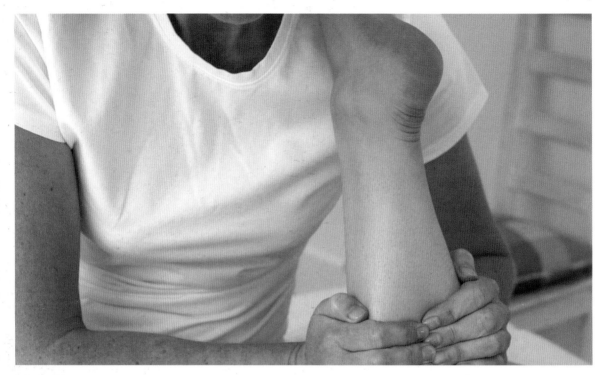

15 **Wrap your hands around the calf** and place the pads of your fingers down the centre of the muscle. Starting just above the heel, apply pressure through your fingers and push them down towards the knee. Repeat and follow with effleurage.

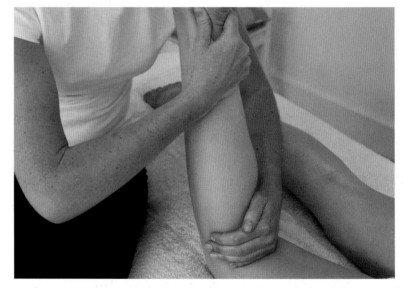

CIRCULAR FRICTION ON ACHILLES TENDON

16 **Support the calf behind the knee** with one hand whilst massaging up either side of the Achilles tendon with small circular moves using the thumb and fingers of your other hand. Do not apply too much pressure as this could cause irritation. Finish with effleurage and gently lower the leg. Repeat steps 11–18 on the recipient's other leg.

Now hold the towel in place and ask your recipient to turn over. Apply the techniques in steps 11–13 to the large muscles at the front of the thigh (known as the quadriceps).

CALF MASSAGE

17 **Support the ankle with your left hand** whilst you effleurage up the fleshy area of the shin with your right hand.

Repeat with small moves from the ankle to the knee – as if you are trying to push the muscle away and down from the shin. Follow with effleurage.

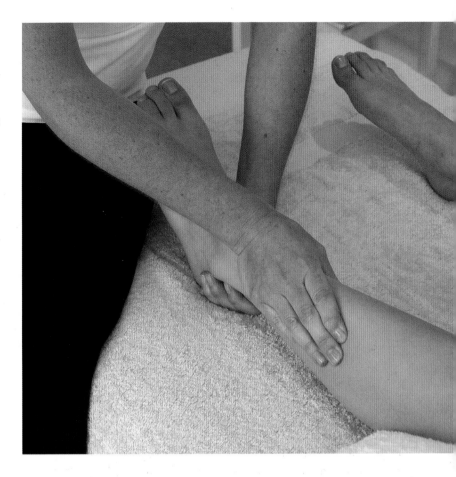

FOOT MASSAGE

18 **Hold the foot in your hands** with your fingers on the sole and your thumbs on the top. Effleurage between the tendons – moving from the base of the toes up to the ankle. Repeat the movement with thumbs working together and alternately.

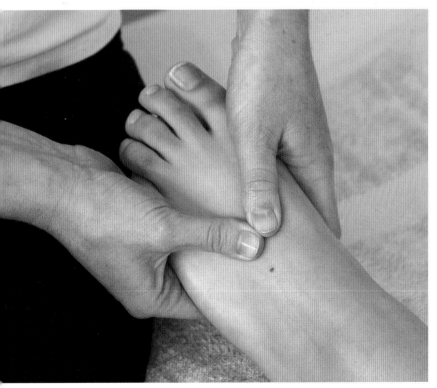

FOOT KNUCKLING

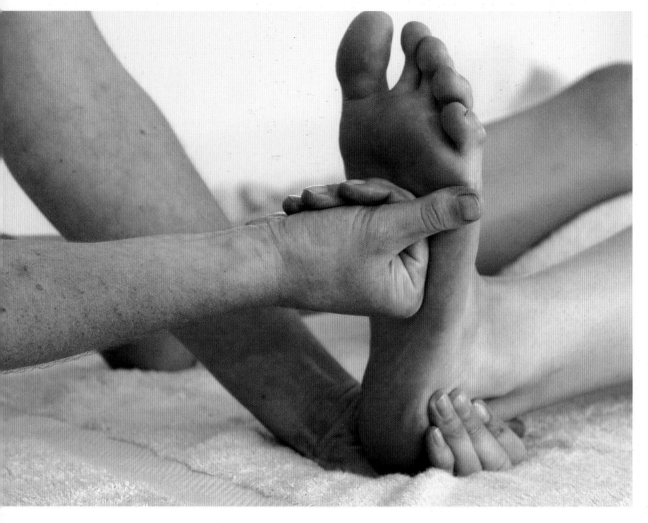

19 **With the foot still resting in your left hand,** try to stretch the calf muscle by pulling your hand toward you. Make a fist with the other hand and massage down from the ball of the foot to the heel. Repeat this action with a rippling/circular movement.

Finish the leg massage with a long effleurage stroke sweeping from the top of the foot up to the top of the thigh.

Repeat steps 19–21 on the other leg.

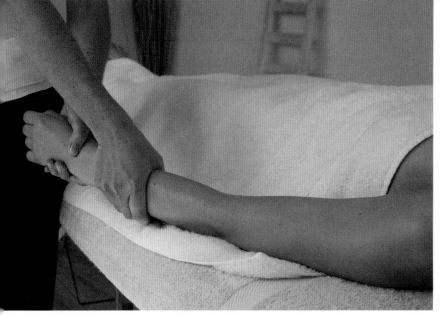

ARM EFFLEURAGE

20 **Standing or sitting about level with the mid-thigh,** hold your recipient's wrist with your hand to support the forearm. Effleurage the arm from the wrist to the shoulder. Try to wrap your hand around the forearm and effleurage up to the elbow then open your hand to stroke up from the elbow to and around the shoulder. Allow your hand to mould into the arm muscles and make sure that you cover all areas. Pull your hand back down under the shoulder and arm to return to the wrist. This pulling back movement should feel like a gentle stretch to the recipient. Repeat several times.

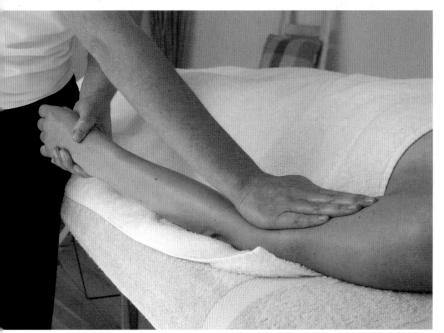

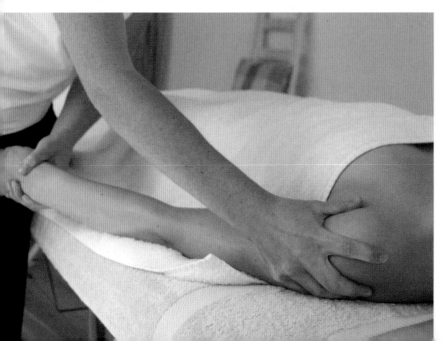

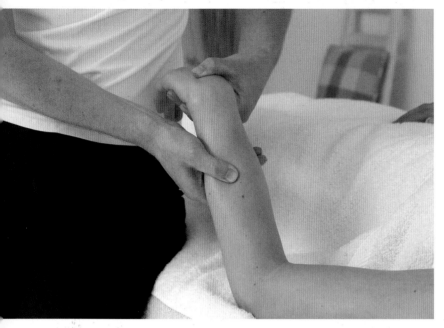

FOREARM FRICTION

21 **Gently bend the recipient's elbow** to lift up the hand. Hold the wrist slightly bent and use the thumb of your other hand to massage up the centre of the forearm. Friction into any areas of tension with your thumbs either stationary, or in small circular or back and forth moves. Finish the arm massage with a long effleurage stroke from wrist to shoulder. Repeat these on the other arm. Place the arms under the towel.

CHEST STRETCH

22 **Stand behind the recipient's head** and place your hands at the base of the neck below the collarbones. Keeping your arms straight, gently push down into your hands to apply a stretch to the chest. Now pull your fingers out across the chest towards the shoulders. When the palms of your hands are on top of the shoulders, with your fingers pointing down the arms, gently push the shoulders down and toward the feet. Repeat this stretch a couple of times.

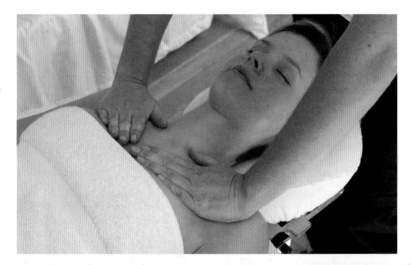

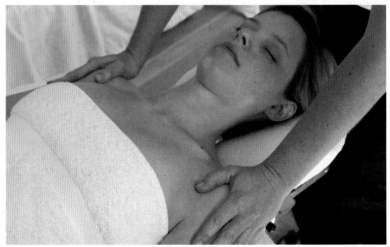

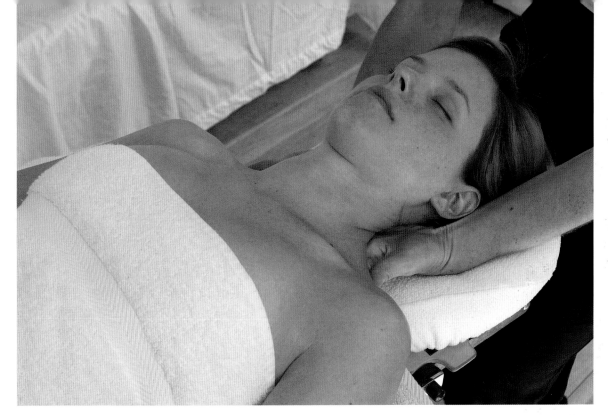

BASE OF THE NECK MASSAGE

23 **Fan your hands under the shoulders** and pull them together and up the base of the neck.

NECK STRETCH

24 **At the base of the neck,** gently raise the pads of your fingers and pull your hands up until your fingers are at the base of the skull. Allow the head to relax on to your fingertips for up to five seconds. Lower your fingertips and return your hands to the base of the neck. Repeat.

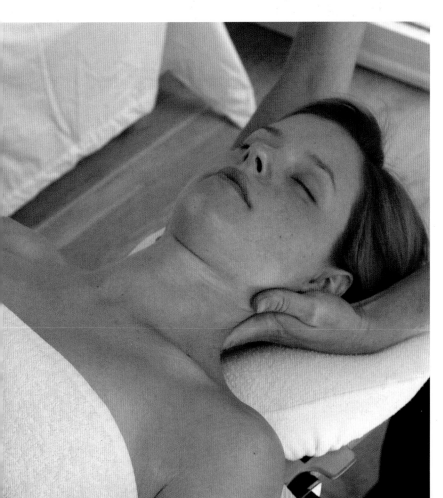

NECK AND SHOULDER MASSAGE

25 **Gently rotate the head to the right** and allow it to rest on your right hand. Wrap your left hand around the left side of the neck, thumb on top and fingers underneath. Slowly effleurage down the neck and across the underside of the shoulder. Still supporting the head with the right hand, cup your left hand around the shoulder and gently stretch the neck by pushing the shoulder down towards the toes. Slowly release the stretch. Repeat.

Slowly return the head to the central position, before rotating it to the left and repeating the above movements.

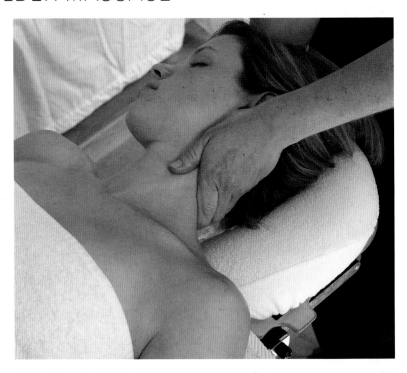

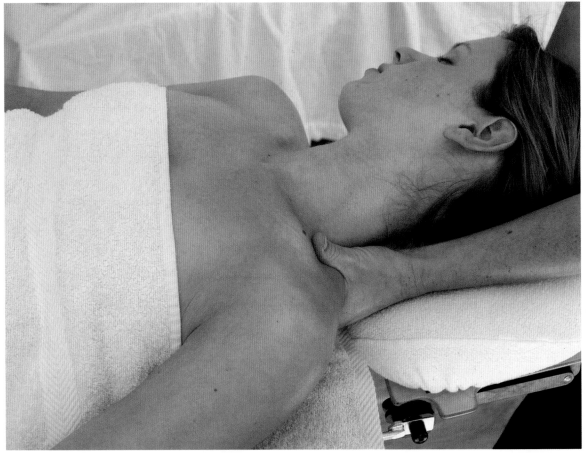

CIRCULAR FRICTION AROUND THE BASE OF THE SKULL

26 **After returning the head to the central position** repeat steps 24–25. At the end of step 25 your fingers should be on either side of the spine at the base of the skull. Apply small circular frictions out towards the ears.

Now spread the pads of your fingers around the base of the skull and gently stretch the neck by leaning your body away from the recipient. Be careful not to raise the recipient's head or overstretch. Release the stretch slowly. Massaging and stretching the base of the skull and the neck will help to relieve headaches and boost the circulation to the head and scalp.

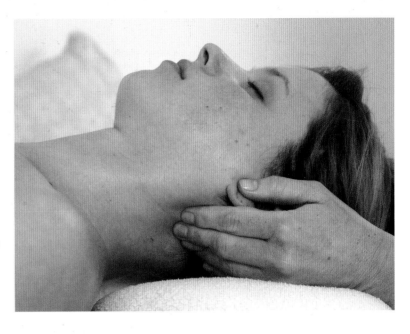

SCALP MASSAGE

27 **To complete the treatment,** pull your fingers up through the hairline to the top of the scalp. Place your thumbs in the centre of the scalp and push the pads of your fingers back down to the hairline and repeat. Finally, place your hands flat on the scalp with your fingers pointing down towards the ears and hold for up to 10 seconds. Gently release your hands from the scalp.

THE PERSON you have massaged will probably need at least a few minutes before they feel ready to get up. Help them to get up if necessary and advise them to drink plenty of water.

2. Face and scalp massage

Massaging the face and scalp will help to release tension and improve circulation, thus toning the skin and hair and helping to impart a youthful glow.

BACKGROUND

The face is our primary organ of expression and acts as a signal of our general health. The muscles in the face reflect our emotions, traumas and stresses, which can often leave a drawn expression, furrowed brows and wrinkles around the eyes and mouth.

The head has 14 facial bones and 22 cranial bones and weighs around 5kg/11lbs. It needs many muscles to hold it in place, elevate the eyebrows, close the eyes, eat, flex, turn and to give expression. Many of these muscles extend down the spine. Tension can restrict the flow of oxygen and blood to the face and will slow the release of toxins through the lymphatic system. This results in the face taking on a taught, dull and sometimes wrinkled appearance and expression.

Tension in the face and scalp not only affects the skin and hair, but can also trigger ailments of the eyes, nose and jaw such as headaches, migraines, sinusitis, skin disorders and jaw grinding. Teeth grinding and clenching are common examples of unconscious stress held in the jaw muscles. Massaging the face and scalp will help to release tension and improve circulation, thus toning the skin and hair and helping to impart a youthful glow.

TECHNIQUE

A professional face and scalp massage will last for approximately one hour. The therapist will take a full case history, including your general health, dietary habits and your home beauty routine. The treatment will take place on a massage couch and the therapist usually uses an oil or cream specifically for the face.

Following all the steps in our guided massage will take approximately one hour. You do not have to stick to a set sequence, but a natural order would be to start on the forehead; then work down to the chin, the ears, the neck and then the scalp. However you choose to give the massage, try to make your sequence flow smoothly and remember how sensitive some areas of the face can be – the eyes, for example.

If you are using oil or cream, use it very sparingly and avoid putting it too near the eyes. Contact lenses should be removed. If you're not using any lubricant, be careful not to drag the skin. Face and scalp massages generally use slow and calming movements. Brisk and fast movements can be added for more stimulation. The recipient should be treated on a massage couch or a suitably padded floor or table. Make sure they are kept warm by a towel or blanket. You should sit on a low stool or kneel, facing the top of the head. As you are going to remain in the same position, it's essential that you are comfortable too.

Look at the face of the person you are going to treat. Do they want a face and scalp massage purely for relaxation or are they suffering from sinus problems, headaches, jaw locking or teeth grinding? Does their skin look lined and tired? These questions will help you to pinpoint the areas of tension in their face and scalp, which will need the most attention during the treatment.

Before you start the guided massage, you should have run through the list of contraindications on page 10–11 with the person you are going to treat. If you are both confident that there is no reason why the treatment should not be given, you can begin.

Massaging around the eyes helps to treat eyestrain, circling the temples soothes headaches and massaging down the nose and along the cheekbones unblocks congestion and sinusitus.

BENEFITS

Facial massage helps to improve skin tone and promote healthier hair, as well as giving a powerful sense of wellbeing. Face and scalp massage can also be used to treat chronic headaches, jaw stiffness, insomnia and sinus problems.

STARTING THE FACE MASSAGE

1 **Stand or sit at the head of your recipient** and place your warmed hands on their head. Your thumbs should be together in the centre with your fingers down the side of the head and over the temples. Hold your hands in this position for up to 10 seconds, relaxing and focusing on your breathing. This will help both you and your recipient to relax.

If you are going to use oil or cream, apply it to your hands now and gently stroke up the base of the neck to the cheeks, up and down the nose, across the cheekbones and up to the temples, finishing with your hands in the centre of the forehead.

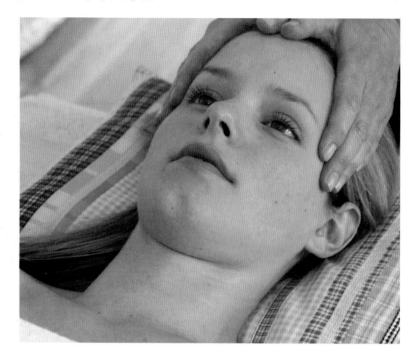

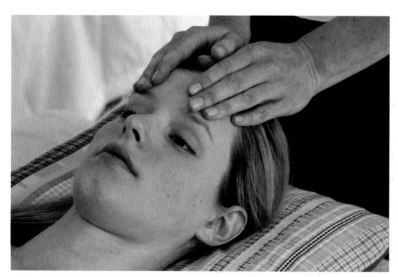

FOREHEAD EFFLEURAGE

2 **Starting from this position,** slowly effleurage out across the forehead to the temples. Apply a gentle downward pressure onto the centre of the temples and hold for a couple of seconds.

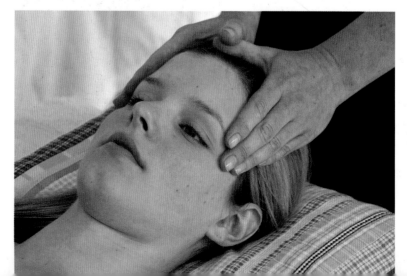

CIRCLING THE TEMPLES

3 **Using the pads of your fingers,** circle the temples clockwise for up to 40 seconds and repeat for 40 seconds in an anti-clockwise direction. Pull your hands back to the centre of the forehead and repeat. This is very soothing for anyone suffering from headaches.

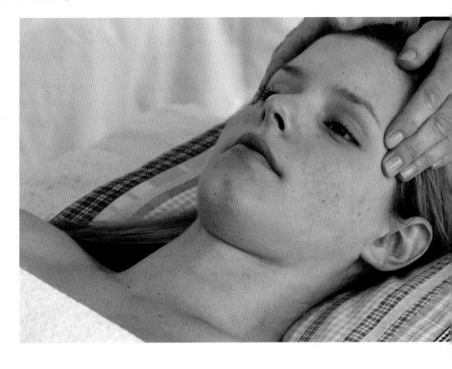

FOREHEAD THUMB CIRCLING

4 **Place the outer border of your thumbs** below the hairline in the centre of the forehead with your fingers pointing towards the ears. Pull the outer border of your thumbs in circular movements towards your fingers. Repeat down the forehead to just above the bridge of the nose.

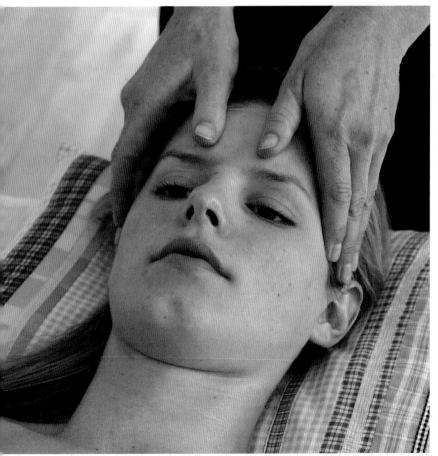

SMOOTHING
THE EYEBROWS

5 **With your index and forefingers,** effleurage out along the eyebrows to the temples, circle under the eyes, pull up the side of the nose and return to the inside edges of the eyebrows.

Press the tips of your forefingers into the bony rim of the eye sockets and hold for 10 seconds. Move to the middle of the eyebrow (directly above the pupil) and hold for 10 seconds. Repeat at the end of the eyebrows and on the temples. Massaging around the eyes is wonderful for relieving eyestrain and tension.

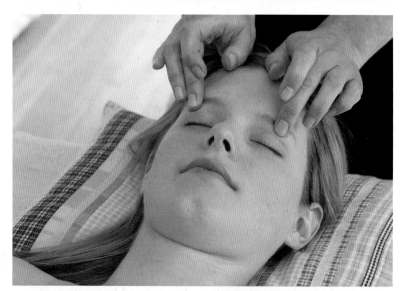

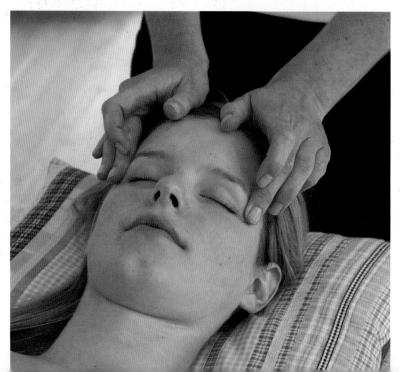

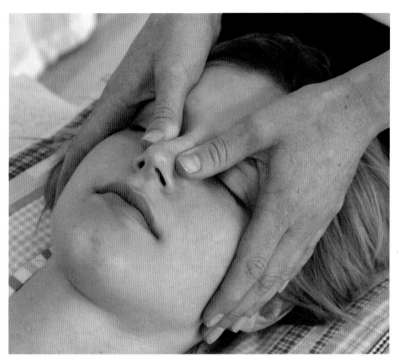

EFFLEURAGING THE NOSE AND CHEEKBONES

6 **Place the outside edge of your thumbs** on the bridge of the nose and effleurage down and out along the base of the cheekbones. Pull your thumbs up and around the eyes and return to the bridge of the nose. Repeat.

Massaging down the nose is helpful for clearing congestion in the sinuses.

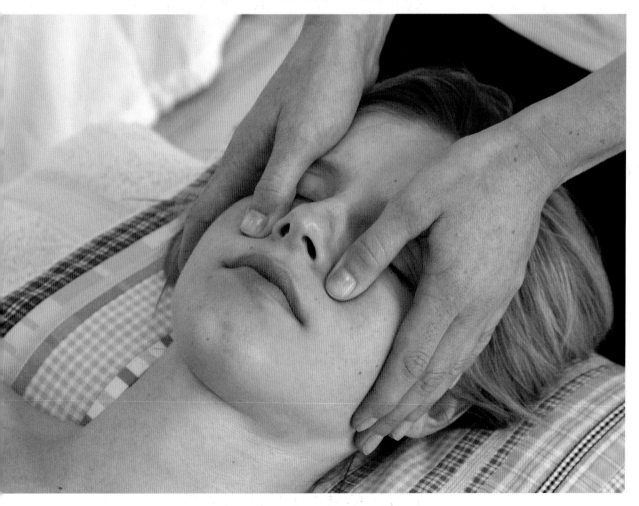

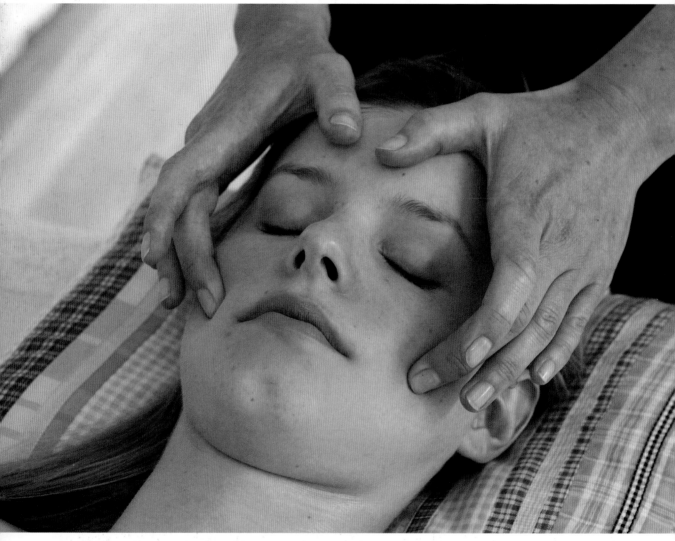

7 **With your thumbs resting on the forehead,** apply pressure to four points along the cheekbones with the pads of your forefingers. The first point is at the junction of the nose and the cheekbone, the second is directly below the pupil, the third point is in line with the end of the eyebrow and the fourth point is at the end of the cheekbone, just before the ear. Press each point for 10 seconds and follow with step 6, effleurage. Repeat.

CHIN AND
JAW MASSAGE

8 **With your thumbs in the centre of the chin** and your index finger under the jaw, effleurage out and around the jaw, reaching up to the ears. Repeat.

Now pinch along the jaw line using your thumbs and the pad of your index fingers. Start in the centre of the chin and work out towards the ears. Follow with effleurage and repeat.

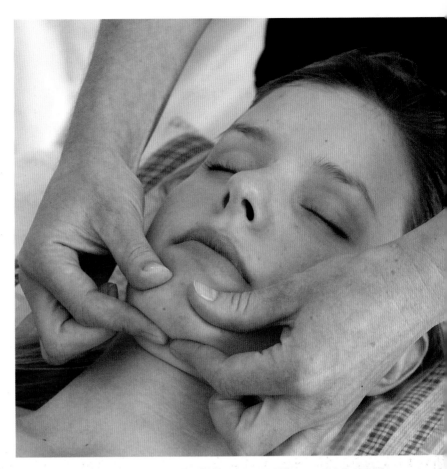

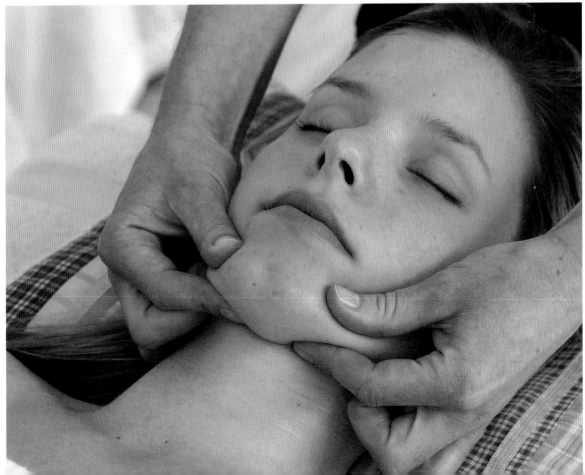

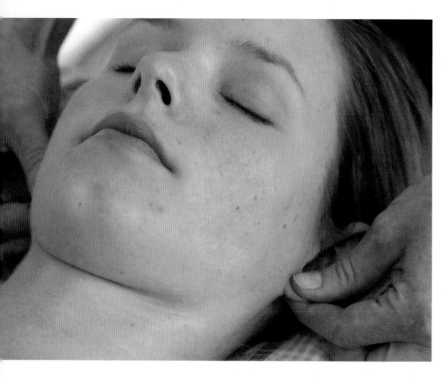

EAR MASSAGE

9 **Grasping the ear lobe** between your forefingers and thumbs, squeeze and gently pull it – moving from the lobe to the top. Now place your forefingers into the ear crevices and follow them back down to the lobe. Repeat.

SCALP MASSAGE

10 **Massage up around behind the ears** with the pads of your fingers and then comb your fingers up through the hair to the top of the scalp. Place your thumbs on top of the scalp and push the pads of your fingers back down. Claw your fingers and thumbs in little circles all over the scalp. Releasing tension here has a great knock-on effect on relaxing the rest of the body.

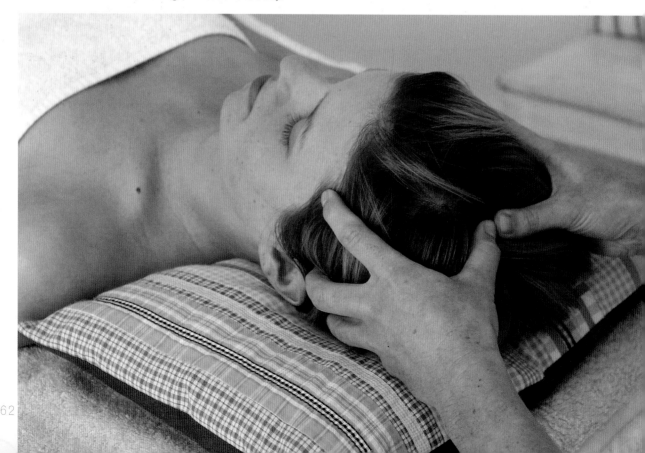

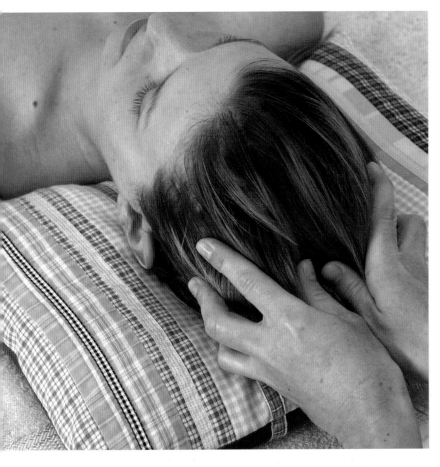

HAIR PULL AND RELEASE

11 **Place the pads of your fingers** around the hairline and pull the hair up and away from the face. Release the hair and repeat.

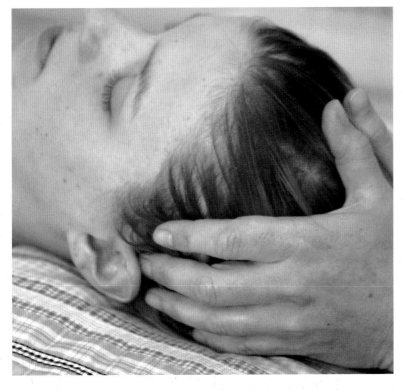

CLOSING RELAXATION

12 **Complete the treatment** by placing your hands on either side of the head with your fingers pointing toward the ears and your thumbs together in the centre. Relax into this position for 40 seconds before gently drawing your hands up and away.

THE PERSON you have massaged will probably need at least a few minutes before they feel ready to get up. Help them up if necessary and advise them to drink plenty of water.

3.Reflexology

Reflexology is the application of pressure over nerve endings in the feet to revitalize and stimulate the body's natural healing powers.

BACKGROUND

Reflexology is the treatment of specific points of the feet. It is based on the theory that every part of the body corresponds to a precise point on the foot and that applying pressure to these points can stimulate the body's natural healing powers to treat minor disorders. In the early twentieth century, Americans Dr William Fitzgerald and Eunice Ingham developed a technique known as "zone therapy", concluding that zones run through the body and that the most effective way of treating them was to work on the feet.

The theory is that the body is divided into 10 zones or energy channels, known as "meridians", with five zones on each side, running from the feet to the head and down the arms to the hands. Every organ and body part lies along one or more of these zones and the foot map is used to locate reflex points. Reflexologists believe that weaknesses in the body can be detected by sensitivity in the corresponding reflex point. By working on these, the body's flow of energy and ability to heal itself will be restored.

The weight of the body can also cause problems in the feet, such as swelling and the collection of calcium crystals. Reflexology helps to boost the circulation and break down these crystalline deposits. It is a great treatment for promoting relaxation and a sense of wellbeing. Each foot contains thousands of nerve endings, making them highly sensitive and responsive.

TECHNIQUE

A professional reflexology treatment will often take place on a specialized reflexology chair, with only the feet exposed. The treatment will last from 45 minutes to an hour. The therapist will take a thorough case history of the client's health and lifestyle. Reflexology is often offered in courses of six treatments, the regularity of which depend upon the condition of the person.

You could give your reflexology treatment on a massage table, a bed or an ordinary chair. However, the feet of the person you are massaging need to be at your chest level, so that you can apply suitable pressure. It's important that you are comfortable too – remember you will be in the same position throughout the treatment.

Following all the steps in the guided treatment will take approximately one hour. Try to make sure that the sequence flows smoothly and apply the techniques with sensitivity – you want to avoid tickling the feet or being too heavy handed. Always support the foot you are massaging by placing one hand around the ankle whilst the other hand applies the techniques. Cover the foot you are not working on with a towel to keep it warm.

Points that are tense or sensitive may signify a blockage and granules under the skin may be waste products such as calcium crystals. However, a tender reflex point does not always mean that there is a problem in the corresponding body organ and you must never attempt to diagnose, unless you are qualified to do so. Slowly increase your pressure to work into these areas to try to break down deposits and eliminate toxins.

When you are ready to start the reflexology, look at the feet of the person you are treating. You may want to give them a quick clean with a wet wipe or similar. Double check for any skin conditions or cuts to avoid. Then warm your hands and start by applying powder into and over the feet. Communicate with the person you are treating throughout the session, to make sure that you aren't causing them discomfort or pain – it will be normal for them to feel a slight tingling sensation.

- **Left and right foot: Left and right side of the body**
- **Toes: Head and neck**
- **Balls of feet: Chest, lung and shoulders**
- **Arch of foot: Diaphragm and waist**
- **Heel: Pelvis**
- **Inner foot: Spine**
- **Outer foot: Arm, shoulder, lower back, hip, leg, knee**
- **Ankle: Reproductive organs**

Before you start the guided massage, you should have run through the list of contraindications on pages 10–11 with the person you are going to treat. If you are both confident that there is no reason why the treatment should not be given, you can begin.

BENEFITS

Reflexology can be effective in cases where an area of the body is traumatized or diseased and direct contact would not be appropriate, and it is also convenient because the recipient doesn't have to be undressed. It improves circulation, helps in the elimination of waste products, revitalizes and induces relaxation.

PREPARING
THE FOOT

1 **Sit or kneel at the feet of your recipient,** with their feet level with your chest. Wipe the feet with a warm cloth, before wrapping your hands around them and holding for up to 10 seconds. Grasp under the ankles and stretch the legs by leaning back. Relaxing and focusing on your breathing during these opening techniques will help both you and your recipient to relax.

Now take one foot between your fingers and your thumbs, with the fingers on the top of the foot and the thumbs on the soles. Squeeze and press the foot all over from the toes to the heel.

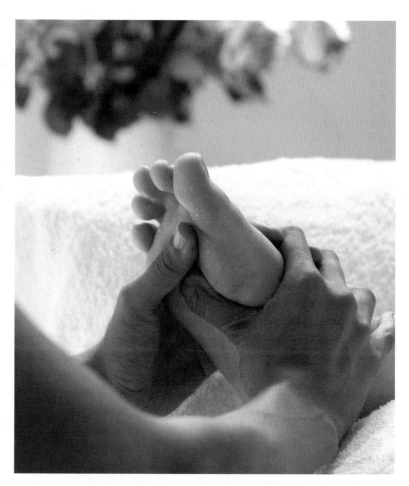

SOLAR PLEXUS
PRESS

2 **With one hand supporting the foot under the ankle,** use the thumb of your other hand to press the solar plexus point of the foot and hold for a couple of seconds. The solar plexus regulates the functioning of the organs and calms the nervous system. To find this point, put your hand on top of the foot and squeeze – the solar plexus point is in the hollow that appears on the sole of the foot. Release slowly.

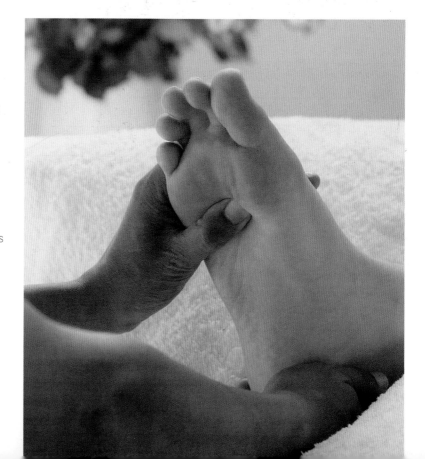

SQUEEZING THE FOOT

3 **Grasp the sole of the foot with your thumbs** and your fingers on the top of the foot. Squeeze and pull up from the heel to the toes. Repeat.

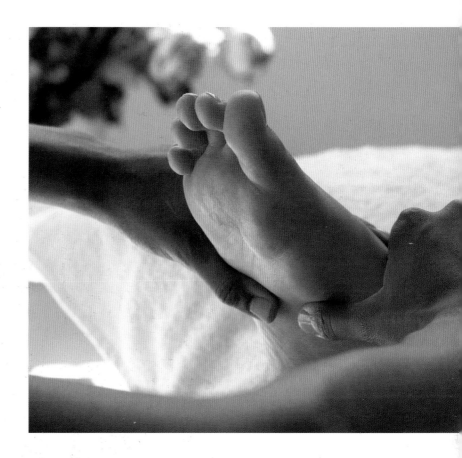

STROKING BETWEEN THE TOES

4 **Holding the foot with one hand,** slide the thumbs of your other hand down between the troughs of the toes on the top of the foot. Repeat each move with thumbs either working together or alternately.

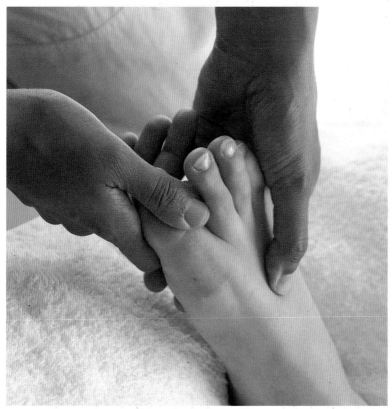

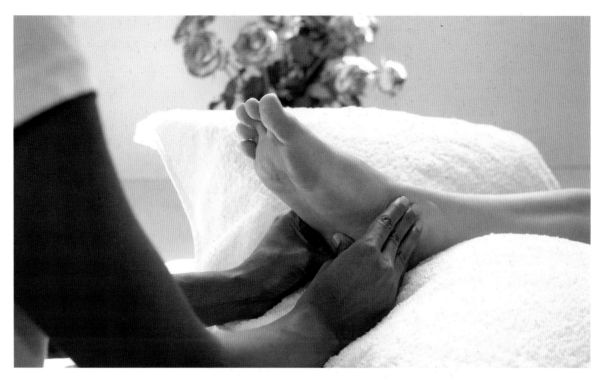

CIRCLING THE ANKLE

5 **Hold the foot with your thumbs on the sole** of the foot and your fingers on the top. Circle the pads of your fingers around the inside and outside of the ankle and up the Achilles tendon. Repeat.

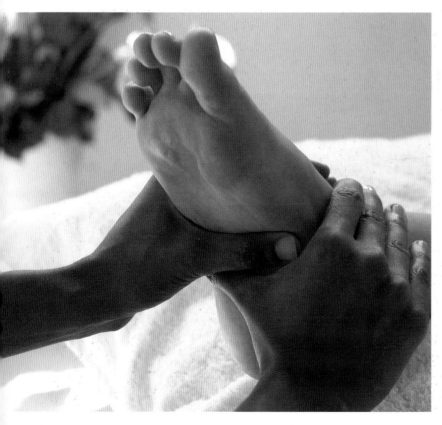

THUMB PRESSURE ON SOLES

6 **Hold the foot with your thumbs on the sole** of the foot and your fingers on the top. Starting on the outside edge of the ball of the foot, press the pads of your thumbs into the foot. Push them towards and past each other to the opposite side and then pull them back to the edge of the foot. Repeat this criss-crossing action down the soles of the foot to the heel and then work back up to the toes. Applying pressure to the solar plexus point on the foot regulates the functioning of the organs and calms the nervous system, thereby relaxing the recipient.

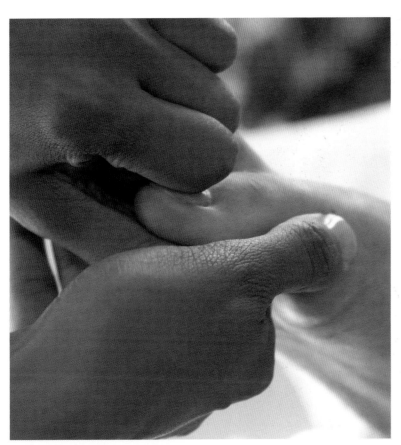

CATERPILLAR DOWN THE THE FOOT

7 **Support the foot by cupping it in the palm of your hand** and place the thumb of your other hand on the outside edge of the big toe. Now walk your thumb like a caterpillar down to the outside edge of the foot to the heel. Effleurage up around the ankle bone. Swap hands and repeat the above movements on the other edge of the foot.

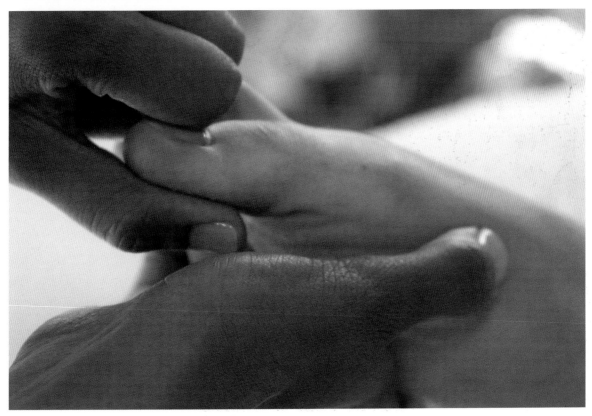

SOLE MASSAGE

9 **Grasp the toes and the top of the foot** between your fingers and thumb. Make a fist with your other hand and press the back of the fingers into the ball of the foot. Slide your fist down the sole of the foot towards the heel. Your supporting hand should move down the top of the foot towards the heel at the same time. Repeat.

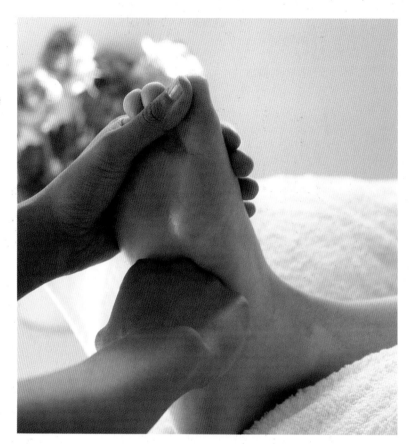

TOE STRETCH

10 **Hold the big toe between your thumb** and forefinger and gently pull it to create a stretch. Release the stretch and, keeping your fingers in the same position, rotate the toe clockwise and then anti-clockwise. Release and repeat on every toe.

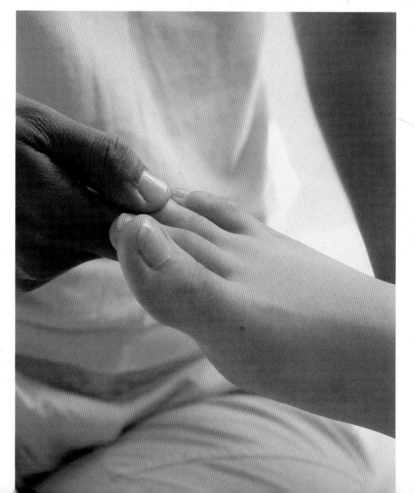

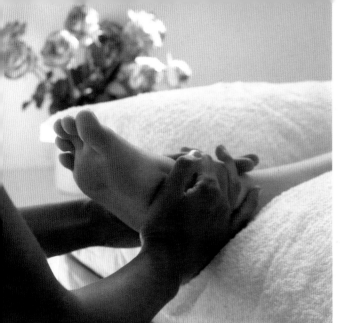

FOOT EFFLEURAGE

11 **Place both of your hands on the top of the foot** and effleurage from the toes up to the ankles. Rotate your fingers around the ankles and pull your hands up and under the heel to return up the base of the foot. Repeat.

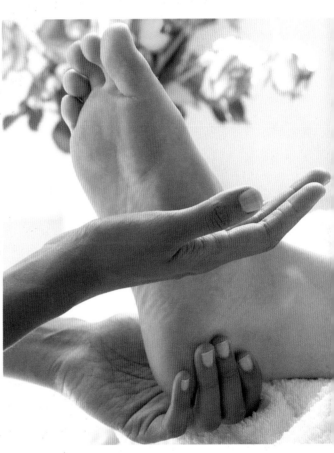

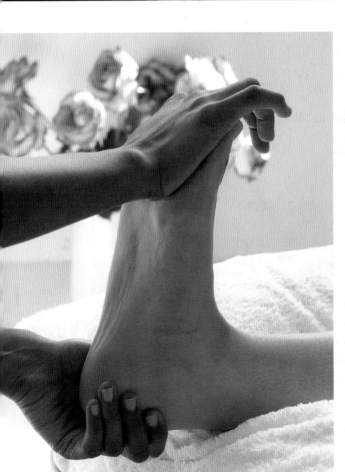

HACKING

13 **With the foot still resting in the cup of your hand,** apply a single-handed hacking up and down the sole of the foot.

Finish the reflexology session by sweeping your hands down the top and base of the foot from the ankle to the toes. Wrap your hands around the foot and hold for 10 seconds, before covering it with a towel. Repeat all the steps on the other foot.

THE PERSON you have massaged will probably need at least a few minutes before they feel ready to get up. Help them to get up if necessary and advise them to drink plenty of water.

ACHILLES STRETCH

12 **Cup the heel of the foot in one hand** and with the other, press forward on the ball of the foot. Now gently pull the heel of the foot towards you – hold for 10 seconds and release.

4. Pregnancy massage

Massage can soothe some of the aches and pains of pregnancy and help a woman deal with the hormonal changes that are occurring in her body.

BACKGROUND

In Africa, India and many other parts of the world, massage has been used for thousands of years to increase fertility and aid childbirth. In the East, it is traditional for a new mother to be pampered after childbirth and every 40 days she will be given a full body massage from a midwife to help ease the aches of childbirth and the anxiety of motherhood.

Prenatal massage has now grown in popularity in the West with the recognition of its therapeutic value. Pregnancy is a time when a woman's focus will be very much on her body, its structural changes and the growth of her baby. The body adapts itself to its increasing burden, but these changes are often accompanied by discomfort, strain and swelling. Massage can help soothe these aches and pains and help a woman deal with the hormonal changes occurring in her body.

It is advisable that the individual check with her doctor before receiving a treatment. Massage is not recommended during the first trimester, and when giving a foot massage, pressure must never be applied to the area between the ankle bone and heel as this area is considered by many therapists to promote early labour. Massage can be used during labour; stroking the face between contractions is calming and reassuring, and massaging the foot helps to alleviate the pain of the contractions.

TECHNIQUE

A professional prenatal massage lasts for approximately an hour or 90 minutes. The therapist will take a thorough case history. A special couch with a supportive hole for the stomach is best for prenatal massage, but an ordinary massage couch can also be used provided the woman's body is positioned and supported correctly. Prenatal massage once a week during the second trimester and twice a week during the third trimester can be highly beneficial.

You can do your guided massage on a massage table, on a suitably padded floor or astride a padded chair. Whichever way you choose, the key is to ensure that the recipient is comfortable and warm and that her body is adequately supported. Place a pillow under her knees to relax the abdomen, and when she

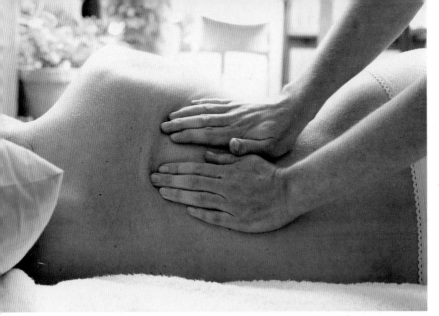

BACK MASSAGE

5 **To effleurage the back in a lying position,** ask your recipient to lie on their left-hand side (lying on the left side during pregnancy can prevent putting the extra weight of the engorged heart on the lungs). Place a pillow under her head and under the uppermost knee, which should be bent at 90 degrees. Massage the back and shoulders following the techniques in steps 1–4.

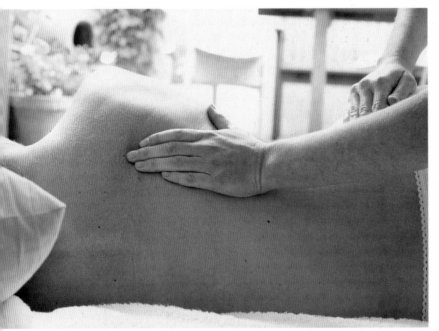

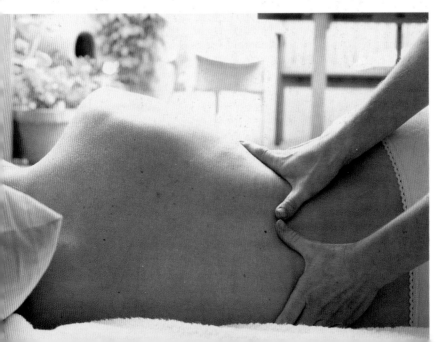

THIGH
EFFLEURAGE

6 **Ask your recipient to slowly lie down on their back,** and cover her with a towel (unless she feels comfortable and warm without one). Place a pillow under the knees. Stand or kneel at the feet of your recipient. Apply a long effleurage stroke from just above the knee to the top of the thigh.

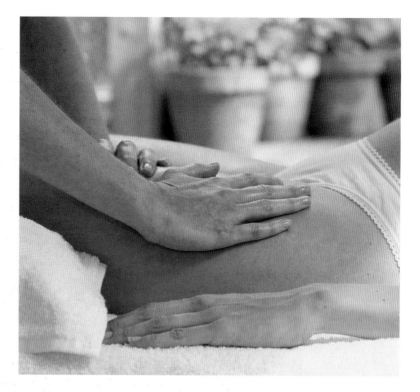

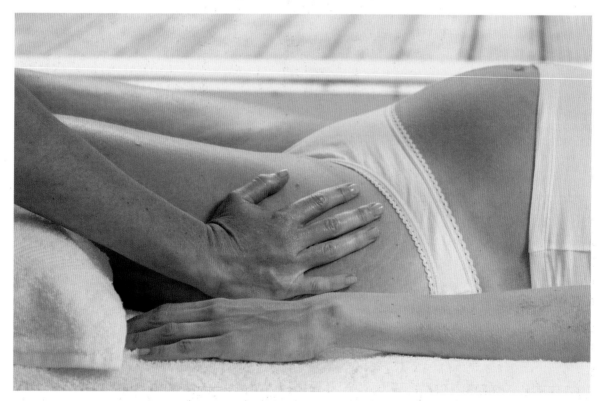

FANNING AROUND THE THIGH

7 **At the top of the thigh, fan your hands out** and sweep them down the inside and outside edges of the thigh.

THIG RING

Kneeling or standing at your recipient's side, place your hands on either side of their lower thigh with fingers pointing away from you and pull one hand towards you as you push the other hand away. Repeat this criss-crossing movement from the knee to the top of the thigh. Repeat and follow with effleurage. You can also knead the legs concentrating on any fleshy or swollen areas. Always follow with effleurage.

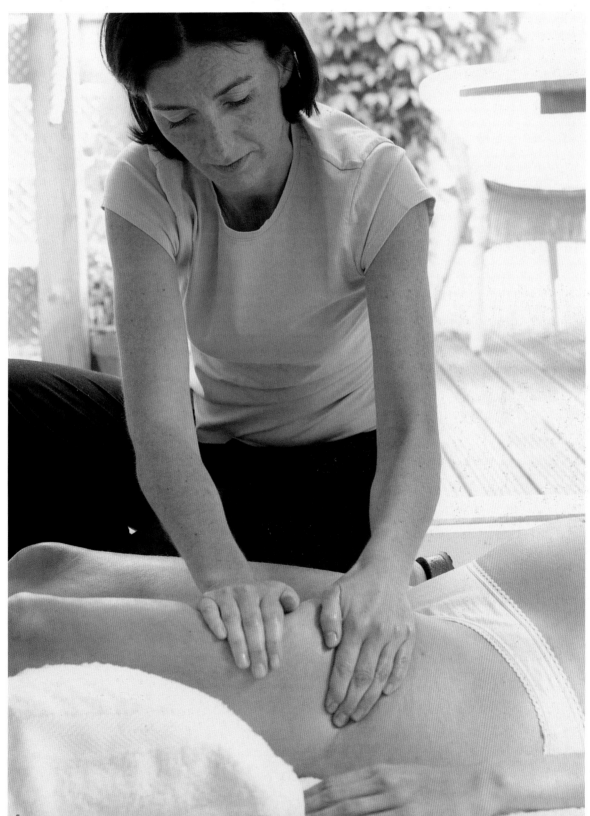

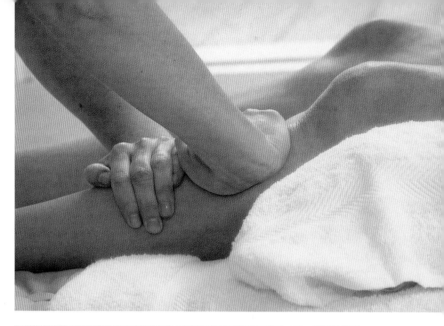

EFFLEURAGING UP THE CALF TO THE THIGH

9 **Kneeling or standing at the recipient's feet,** effleurage from the top of the feet over the knees and up to the top of the thigh. Fan your hands down either side of the thigh and draw them back under the leg to the ankle. Repeat. Always release any pressure as you move over or under the knee.

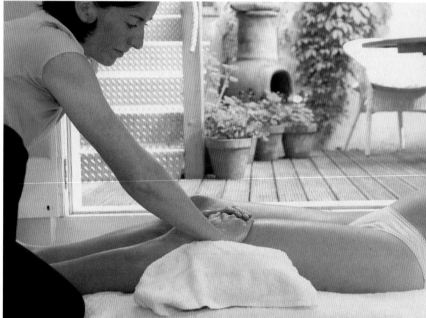

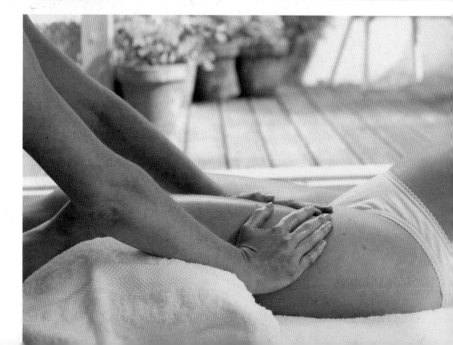

SQUEEZING THE CALF MUSCLES

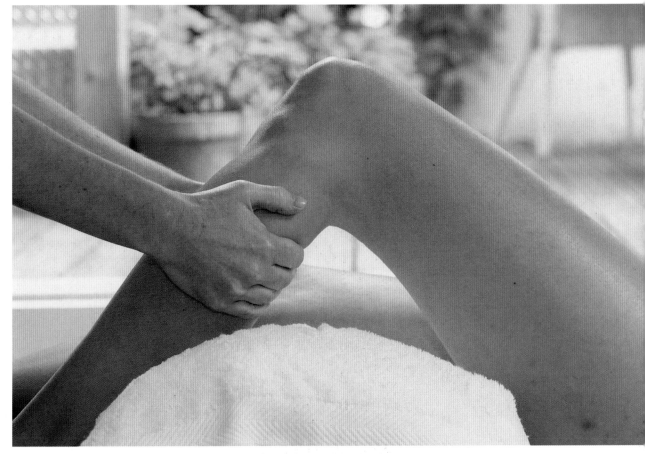

10 **Place one hand under the recipient's knee** and, holding the ankle with your other hand, bend the knee to raise the calf. Hold the foot in place by sitting lightly on or next to it. Place your fingers in the middle of the back of their calf and split the muscle by pulling your fingers towards you. Repeat, moving your hands down the calf to the ankle. Carefully lower the leg back down to the table and follow with an effleurage stroke from just below the knee to the heel.

ANKLE MASSAGE

11 **With the leg flat, effleurage around the ankle in a clockwise direction.** Repeat a couple of circles. Follow with effleurage from the top of the ankle to the top of the thigh and bring your hands back down. Repeat.

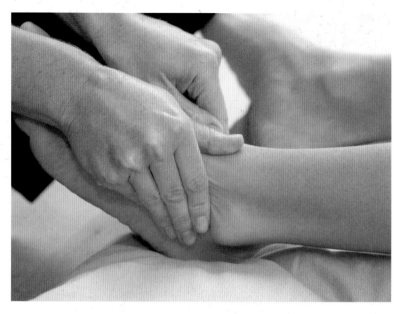

CALF STRETCH

12 **Cup the heel of the recipient's foot** in your hand. With the palm of your other hand on the ball of the foot, pull the heel towards you as you push the ball of the foot away from you. Hold for up to 30 seconds, release and repeat. Cover the leg and foot with a towel and repeat steps 6–13 on the other leg.

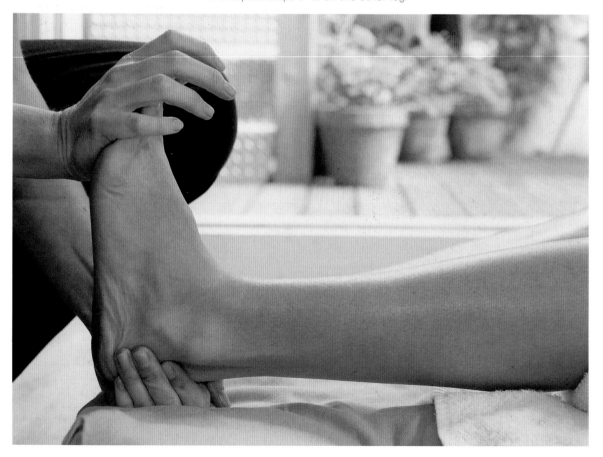

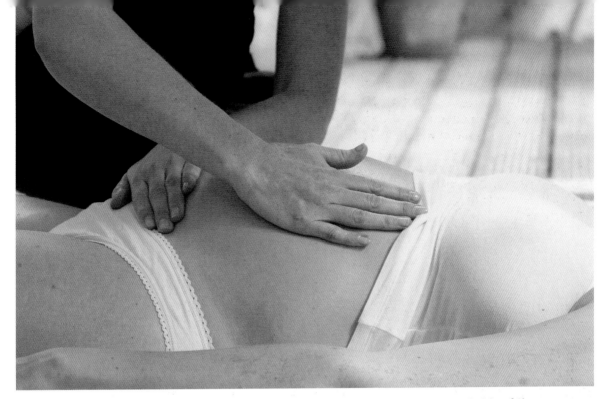

ABDOMEN MASSAGE

13 **Standing or kneeling on the right-hand side of the recipient,** start at the base of the stomach and gently draw your hands across to the right-hand side and then stroke up and around the abdomen in a clockwise direction. Try to use your hands alternately with one following the other – you will be able to make a full circle with one and half a circle with the other, lifting one hand as it crosses the other.

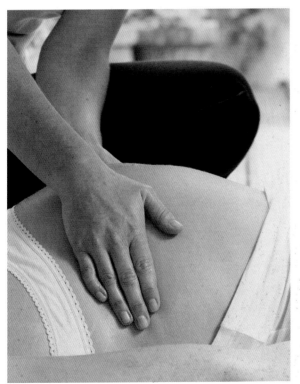

FINISHING STROKES

14 **Place your hands on either side of the waist** and gently draw them up to the navel, slowly lifting them off. Repeat.

THE WOMAN you have massaged will probably need at least a few minutes before they feel ready to get up. Help them off the couch if necessary and advise them to drink plenty of water.

5.Infant massage

Babies receiving regular massages may be less prone to complaints and infections, and may benefit from improved co-ordination.

BACKGROUND

In many countries and cultures, infant massage is an ancient and natural tradition, but it is only since the 1980s that many in the West have also started to recognize its benefits. Regular massage is believed to be an important factor in promoting a child's good health and wellbeing. There is some evidence that babies receiving regular massages are subject to less complaints and infections, and may benefit from improved co-ordination. Massage is a wonderful way of showing love and encouraging a strong bond between parent and child. It can also help develop confident parenting skills and can soothe symptoms caused by minor ailments.

Babies can be massaged very gently from one week after birth throughout childhood. Making massage a nightly or daily occurrence will help a child to recognize routine – after a bath and before bed is an ideal time. Massage can also be effective for calming excited toddlers, but remember that the attention span of a baby or young child is usually very short, so to make the experience most enjoyable for both parent and child, massages should be no longer than 10 to 15 minutes.

TECHNIQUE

Courses are now readily available where parents can go along with their babies or toddlers and learn infant massage from a professional. Often the massage is taught in small groups, so it is quite fun and sociable. If you have any worries or concerns, seek advice from your doctor or health visitor.

You can do your massage on the floor on a changing mat/towel or with the baby lying across your legs. Do be aware that babies often empty their bladder whilst being massaged! Choose a light vegetable oil such as sweet almond oil or sunflower oil – don't use baby oil, as the skin does not easily absorb it.

Following all the steps in the guided massage should take approximately 10 minutes. Don't massage your baby straight after a feed or if he or she may be hungry or too tired.

Make sure the room is a suitable temperature because babies lose heat quickly, so a warm room and hands are essential. Remember to remove any jewellery that could scratch you child.

Starting a massage with your baby lying on its back will allow for eye contact and help your baby feel secure. You could begin with the face and gently massage down to the toes with finger and thumb strokes. Although the pressure should be light, make sure you are not simply tickling. You don't have to follow a set sequence; adapt your techniques to work with your child's body and concentrate on any areas that are causing a problem, for example, if your baby is suffering constipation or colic, massage the stomach. If he or she has a cold, gently massaging the chest and back can help to loosen any phlegm. With practise, you will start to learn what your baby enjoys and what is calming and soothing.

Before you start the guided massage, consider if any of the contraindications on page 10–11 apply to your baby and use your common sense. Never try to treat a child who is ill without first consulting a suitably qualified medical practitioner. Avoid massaging a child's head until they are at least two years old, as it is an extremely delicate area. Do not use essential oils unless recommended and blended by a professional aromatherapist.

To treat constipation, colic or stomach ache, massage the stomach in a clockwise direction. To treat colds or respiratory conditions, massage the chest and back.

BENEFITS

Infant massage is very calming: it induces relaxation and can help a baby's sleeping pattern. It encourages better feeding and can helps treat colic, diarrhoea and constipation. It can ease respiratory conditions such as asthma, bronchial congestion, coughs and colds.

STROKING
ON THE OIL

1 **Put your baby on a changing matt or padded floor.** Warm a little oil in your hands. Gently place your fingers on your baby's forehead and smooth the oil down the cheeks to the chin, neck, across the shoulders, down the arms and then gently sweep the oil from the torso to the feet.

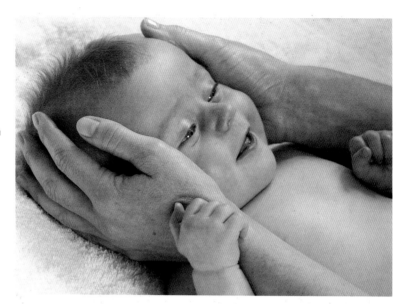

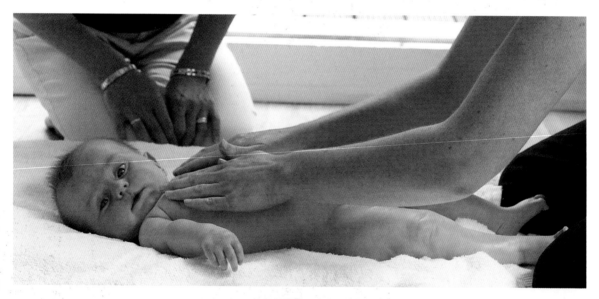

STROKING
ACROSS
THE CHEST

2 **Place your hands on your baby's chest** and fan them out from the centre across the shoulders and down the arms.

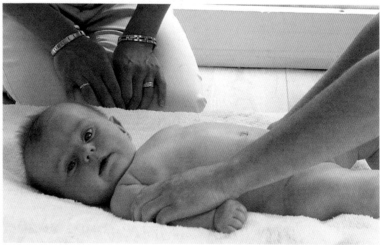

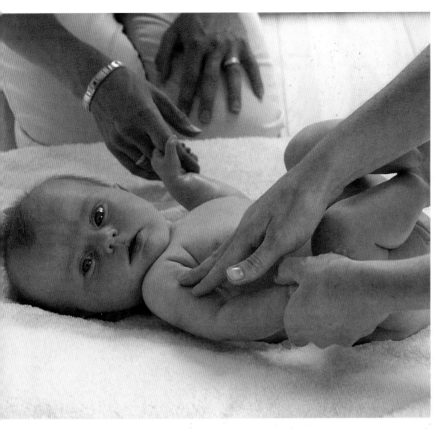

ARM AND HAND MASSAGE

3 **Wrap your fingers around your baby's arm** and with one hand following the other, stroke down your baby's arm to the hand. Massage in and around the hand and gently squeeze down and off each finger. Repeat and then repeat on the other arm.

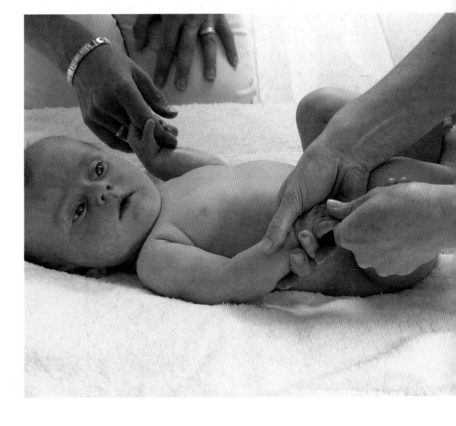

STROKING DOWN THE CHEST

4 **With a gentle feathery stroke,** massage alternately with one hand moving down after the other from the centre of the chest to the top of the abdomen. Repeat a couple of times.

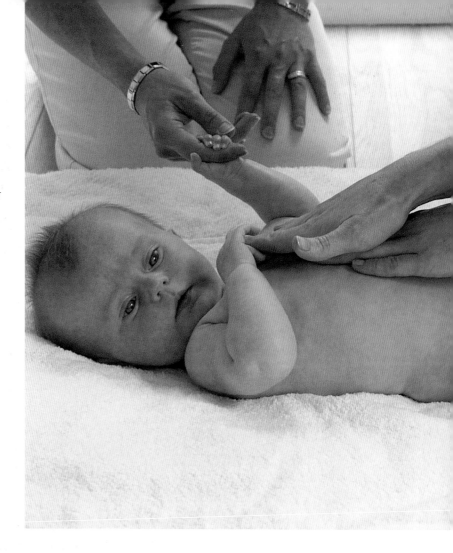

ABDOMEN MASSAGE

5 **With one hand following the other,** stroke your hand around the abdomen in a clockwise direction. You will have to lift one hand as your arms cross each other. Repeat a couple of times or more, if your baby is suffering from constipation or colic. Now place your fingers on either side of the waist and lightly draw your fingers up to the navel to lift off. Repeat a couple of times.

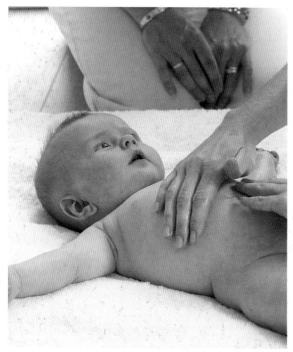

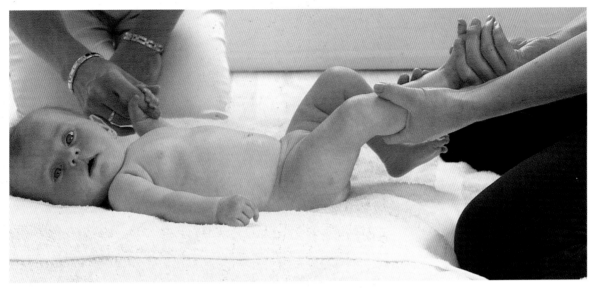

LEG MASSAGE

6 **Wrap your hand around your baby's thigh** and pull down the thigh to the foot, sweep over the foot and pull off at the toes. Before you pull your hand away from the toes, start the movement at the top of the thigh again with your other hand. Repeat a couple of times, and repeat on the other leg.

Effleurage your hands up the front of your baby's legs and torso to the shoulders. Wrap your fingers under the shoulders and massage across the arms. Raise the arms and pull up to the fingers.

BACK MASSAGE

7 **Turn your baby over onto their front** and, if you need to, apply a little more oil to your hands. Pull your fingers down to your baby's lower back and effleurage back up to the shoulders.

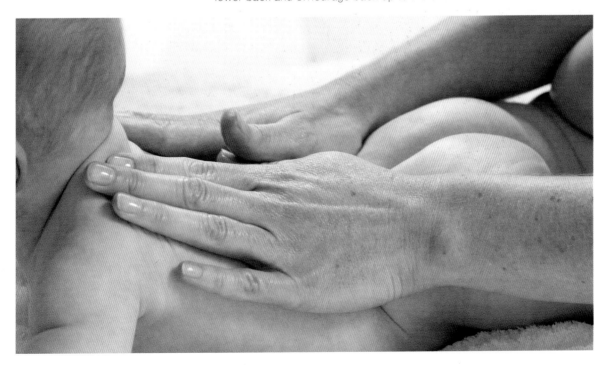

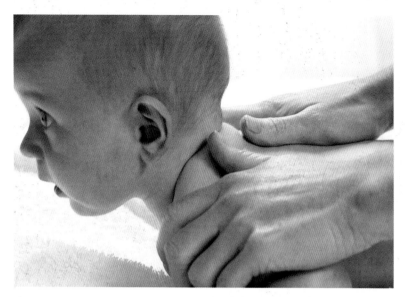

SHOULDER MASSAGE

8 **Gently squeeze the shoulder muscles** between your fingers and thumbs from the neck/shoulder junction to the top of the arms. Repeat.

ARM SQUEEZE

9 **Wrap your fingers around your baby's arms** and stroke and squeeze down to the wrists and through the hands. If your baby's head and neck are in the air, ensure that you do not take the elbows off the mat. You should massage in such a way that the baby does not have to move or lose its balance.

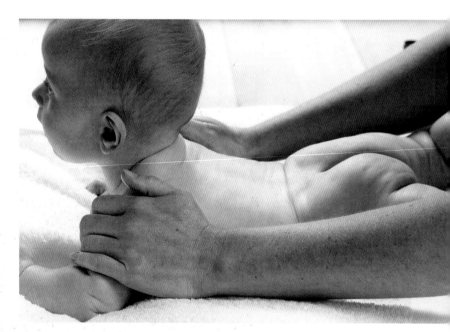

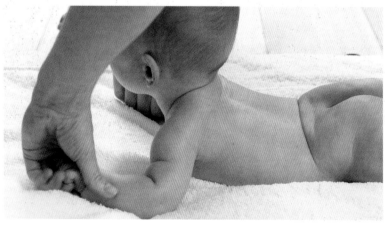

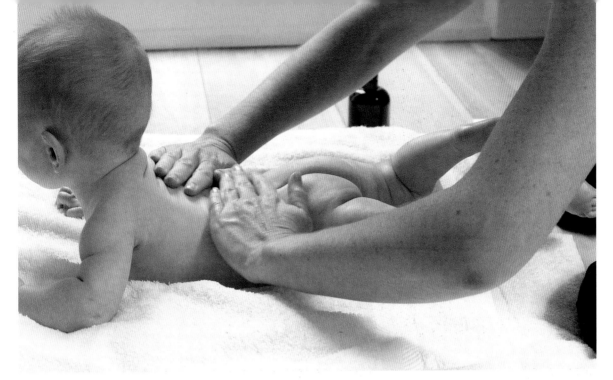

BACK MASSAGE   10 **Return to the top of the back** and alternately pull your fingers down to the buttocks.

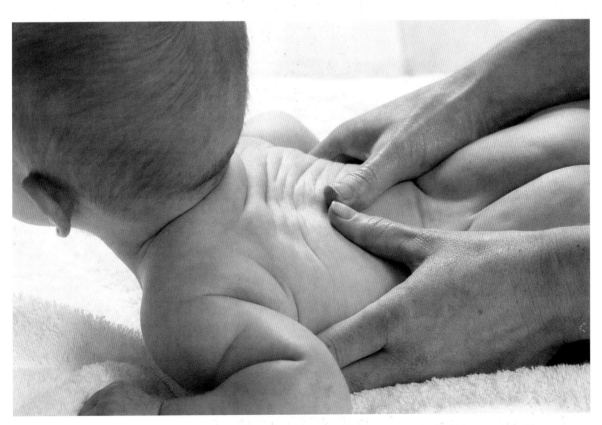

11 **Wrap your hands around your baby's torso** and with your thumbs on either side of the spine, slowly massage up to the neck.

LEG MASSAGE

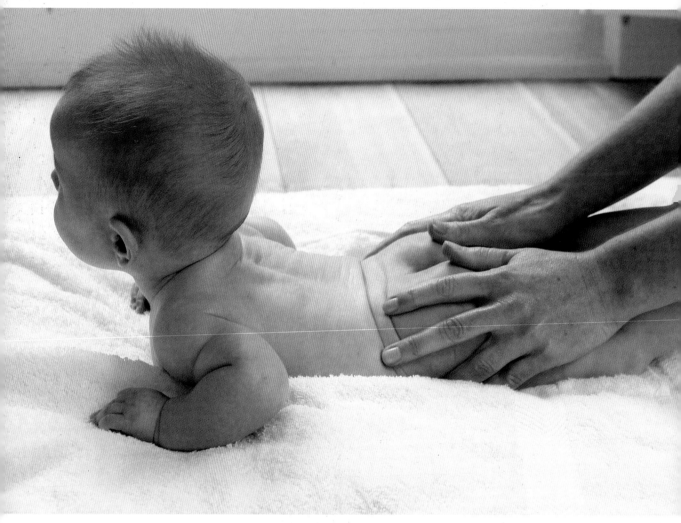

12 **Feather your fingers back down your baby's spine** and massage over the buttocks. Now wrap your fingers and thumbs around the thighs and pull and squeeze your hands from the top of the thighs to the ankles. Wrap your fingers around the foot, raise the legs and do little thumb circles all over the soles of the feet.

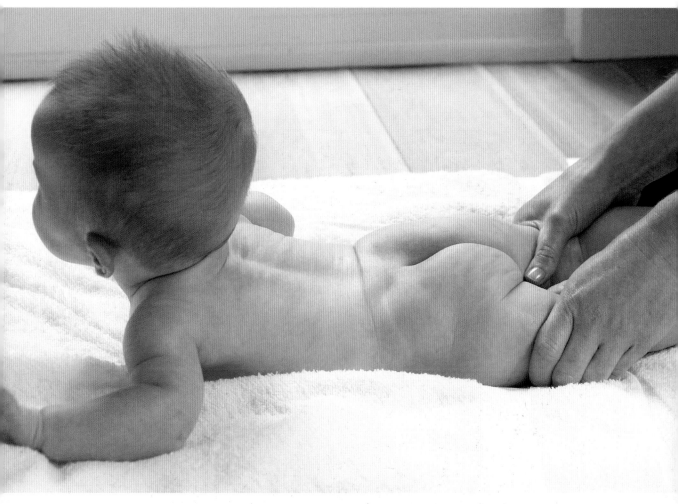

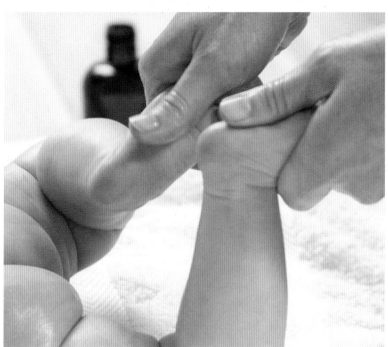

FINISH the massage by gently squeezing each toe. Repeat the squeeze a couple of times before wrapping your baby up in a warm towel for a cuddle.

6. Sports massage (deep tissue massage)

Sports massage is a common means of treating musculo-skeletal disorders and can be performed on the full body or tailored to treat a specific area or injury.

BACKGROUND

Sports and deep tissue massage techniques have been a common means of treating musculo-skeletal disorders for generations. They are used to aid recovery from muscular fatigue, to aid in monitoring the condition of muscle tissues, to treat minor soft tissue injuries and to help enhance muscle performance.

Muscles work in pairs – as one contracts, its partner relaxes – and if one muscle is tense, the opposing muscle has to take additional load, resulting in imbalance and potential injury. Most sports or dance injuries are usually due to postural imbalance or unusual technique. The techniques used are similar to those used in Swedish massage: effleurage, petrissage and friction. Deep tissue and soft tissue manipulation techniques are also used to relax, stretch and strengthen the muscles. The latter techniques require advanced training and a thorough understanding of anatomy and physiology.

Pre-exercise massage aims to stimulate and target specific areas, rather than the full body, and attempts to strike a balance between over stimulation and relaxation. The muscles should not be overworked before an event, but neither should they be allowed to become too relaxed as this will result in loss of power. A deep tissue massage one week before a competition is usually very beneficial.

Post-exercise massage is similar to a warm down and includes plenty of superficial stroking and passive stretching. By stimulating the circulation, the muscles become nourished, which eliminates the waste and swelling that occurs after exercise. A post-exercise massage should be given before stiffness sets in – if it is necessary to wait, the muscles should be kept warm and stretched.

TECHNIQUE

A professional sports or deep tissue massage can treat the full body or be tailored to a specific area or injury. The therapist will take a thorough case history and an anatomical analysis of the client before commencing. Treatments usually take from 30 minutes to an hour and are given on a massage couch. Follow-up treatments and/or home exercises may be recommended depending on the condition of the client.

Our guided massage is not intended to teach the more advanced techniques of sports therapy, but following the steps will help you to relax tightened, restricted muscles in the arms, hands and fingers, thereby improving their flexibility and range of movement. This will help conditions such as carpal tunnel syndrome and tendonitis, which are commonly described under the umbrella term RSI – repetitive strain injury. Many people who regularly work on a computer or carry out other repetitive tasks suffer from these conditions, and poor posture and bad work practices aggravate the strain.

Aligns and supports the musculo-skeletal system, rejuvenates and relaxes muscles and helps regain flexibility and suppleness of the joints.

Being more aware of posture, taking short but frequent breaks from your tasks and regularly following the guided self-massage can help to reduce painful symptoms. Always work on warmed muscles. Do not bounce, hold onto pain or go beyond your pain threshold.

Before you start the guided massage, consider if any of the contraindications on page 10–11 apply to you. If you are confident that there is no reason not to do these techniques, you can begin.

BENEFITS

As well as improved circulation, pain reduction and relaxation, sports massage is effective for injuries such as lower back pain, tennis elbow, sprains, strains and cartilage problems and is a fantastic aid to postural imbalances.

Strains and sprains

Most sports or exercise-related injuries are either strains or sprains. A strain is the tearing of muscle or tendon through over-exertion and results in pain, redness and heat. A sprain occurs when the ligament that supports a joint is torn when pushed beyond its normal range. The symptoms are swelling, bruising and pain with movement or pressure. Try to see a doctor or qualified therapist as soon as possible. Following the steps in Rice and Mice, below, will aid recovery.

RICE (Follow immediately after an injury and continue for up to two days.)

Rest – Movement will aggravate the area and delay healing.

Ice – Apply ice as soon after injury as possible to slow down the swelling. Wrap the ice in a damp cloth or keep it moving over the skin. Do not allow the skin to turn red – if it does you have over iced and may have caused a reverse effect.

Compression – Apply a firm padded strapping to the area to restrict any internal bleeding – but never apply compression to a whole limb.

Elevation – Elevate injured area as often as possible to aid in the removal of swelling.

MICE (Follow 48 hours later when the swelling, heat and redness have reduced.)

Mobilization – Gradually introduce gentle exercise.

Ice – Continue icing until swelling has gone.

Compression – Reduce the compression to a support bandage.

Elevation – Elevate as frequently as possible.

FOREARM AND HAND SELF-HELP

1 **Make a fist with one hand and hold the wrist with your other hand.** The fist hand can either face up or down – try it both ways. Keep the wrist in a neutral position, then slowly lower your fist. As you move it down, resist the movement very gently. Repeat 12 times. Repeat on the other hand. When the power in your wrist improves, try doing this technique with a small weight.

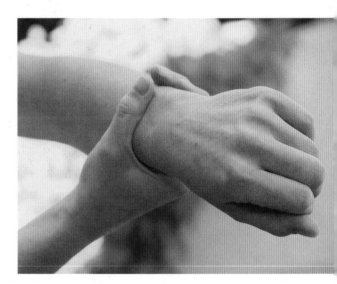

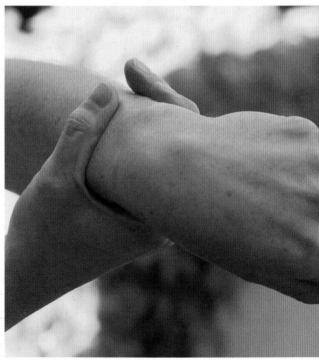

WRIST
ROTATION

2 **Again holding one wrist with the other hand,** move your hand from the wrist in a circle – first clockwise, then anti-clockwise. Repeat on the other hand. Repeat 12 times on each wrist.

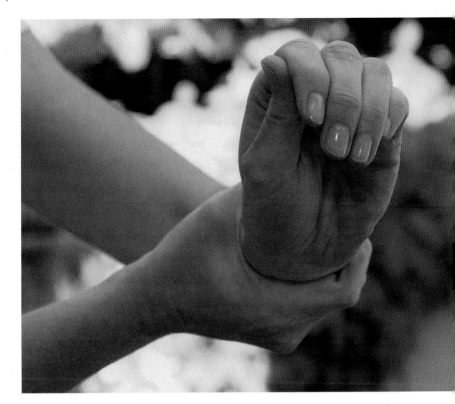

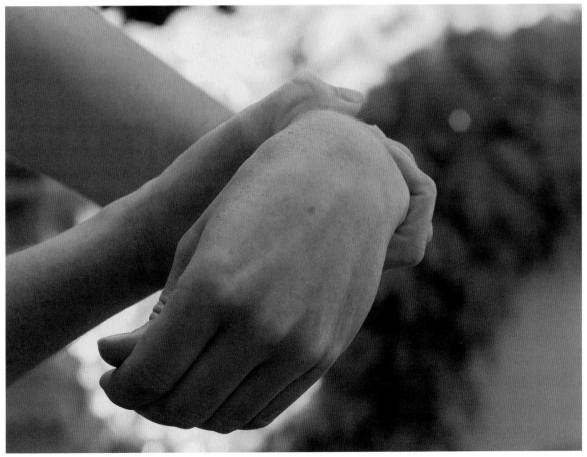

FOREARM FRICTION

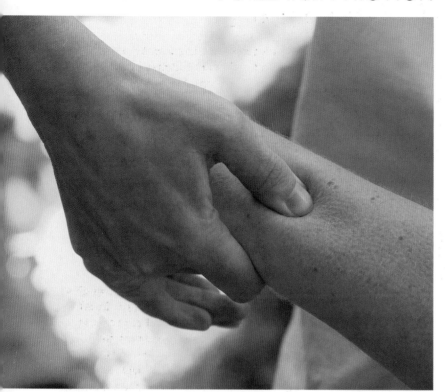

3 **Wrap one hand around your forearm with your fingers** underneath and your thumb on top and stroke your thumb sideways up the forearm muscles, from the wrist to the elbow. Repeat. With your hand in the same position as above, apply stationary pressure to the centre of the forearm with the pad of your thumb. As you apply the pressure, lower your wrist. You should feel a stretch. Do not overstretch or work into pain. Repeat from the wrist to the elbow.

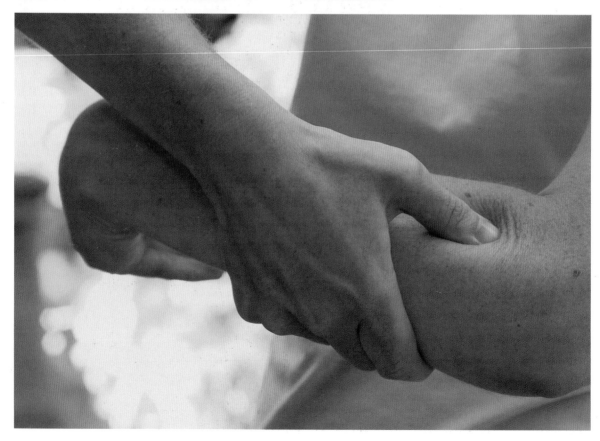

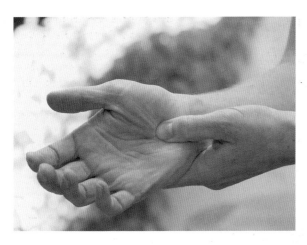

CARPAL TUNNEL MASSAGE

4 **Rest one open hand in the palm of your other hand and friction around the carpal tunnel** with your thumb. The carpal tunnel is the area of your palm through which the tendons and nerves pass into the hand. Applying deep friction around the carpal tunnel on a regular basis can help to prevent injury from repetitive sport or occupational stress. However, do not over-friction, as this can cause irritation and inflammation.

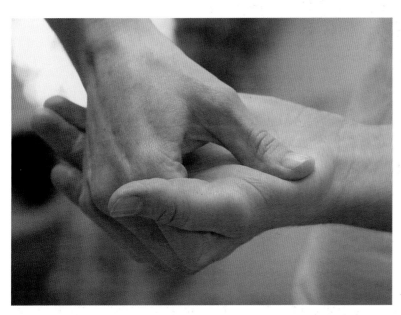

THUMB MASSAGE

5 **Link your thumbs together and rest the upper hand** in the fingers and palm of your lower hand. Friction up and around the muscles of the thumb, concentrating on the thumb/wrist junction, and continue around the palm of the hand.

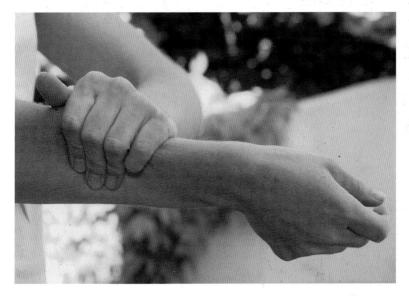

FOREARM SQUEEZE

6 **Wrap one hand around the inside of your forearm** and squeeze the muscles between your palm and fingers, from the wrist to the elbow. Repeat.

FOREARM STRETCH

7 **Standing in front of a chair,** place one hand on the seat with your
fingers pointing towards you and gently lean towards the chair.
Don't lean too far into the stretch and do not use your whole body
weight. Repeat five times, before shaking your hands loosely.

Repeat steps 3–7 on the other hand or arm.

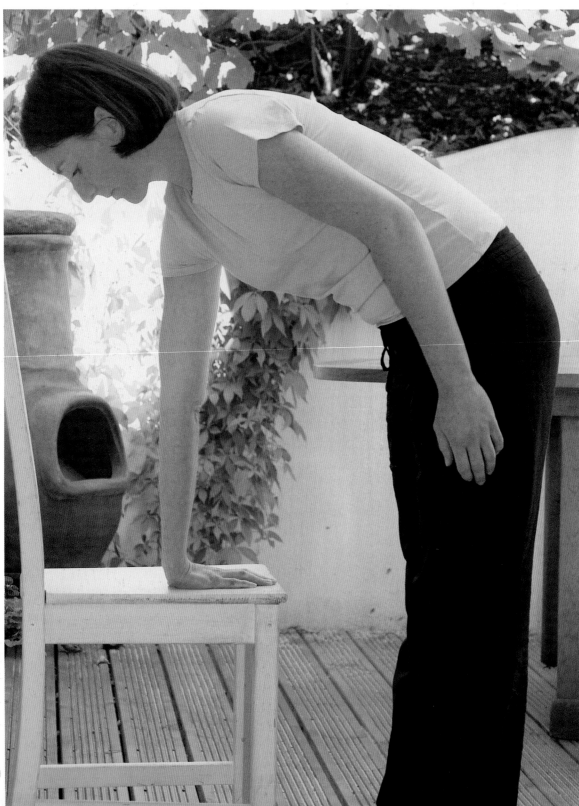

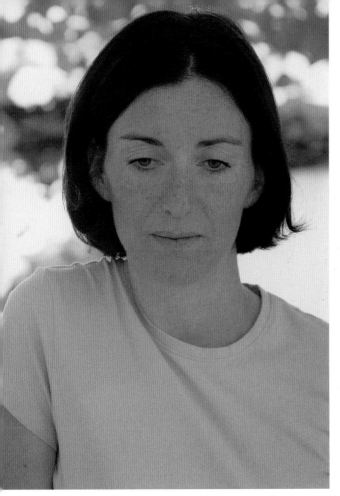

SHOULDER STRETCH

8 **Starting in a neutral position,** slowly raise one shoulder, keeping the arm, neck and back relaxed. Hold for 10 to 15 seconds, return to your neutral position and relax for five seconds. Slowly move your shoulder down, hold for 10 to 15 seconds, return to your neutral position and relax for five seconds. Repeat both stretches five times on each shoulder.

Stretching helps to relax tightened, restricted muscles and improve flexibility and range of movement. Take care to avoid jerky movements, bouncing or going beyond your pain threshold.

NECK STRETCH

9 **Starting in a neutral position,** tilt your head to the right whilst raising your right shoulder a little. Hold for 10 seconds. Return to the neutral position and relax for five seconds. Repeat on the left shoulder. Repeat five times on each shoulder.

Take care to avoid jerky movements, bouncing or going beyond your pain threshold.

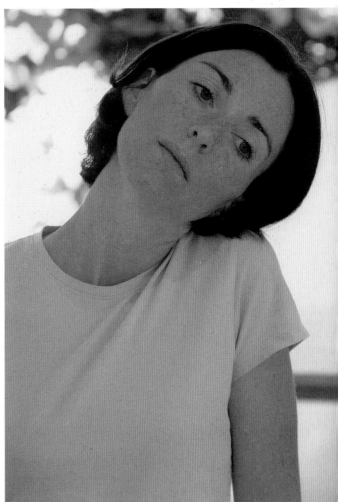

SHOULDER STRETCH

10 **Start in the neutral upright position** and slowly move your shoulder back. Hold for 10 to 15 seconds and move your shoulder back to the neutral position. Relax for five seconds.

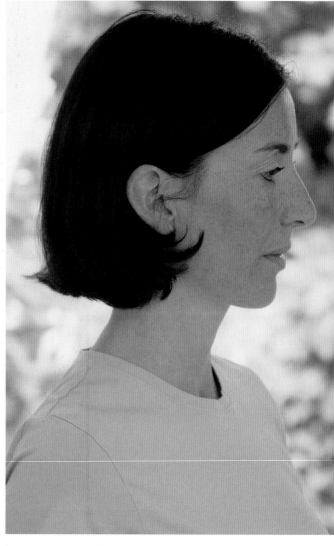

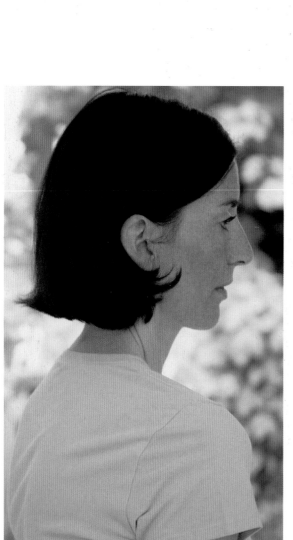

SHOULDER STRETCH CONTINUED

11 **Now slowly move your shoulder forward,** holding it for 10 to 15 seconds, before returning to the neutral position. Relax for five seconds. Repeat five times in both directions with each shoulder.

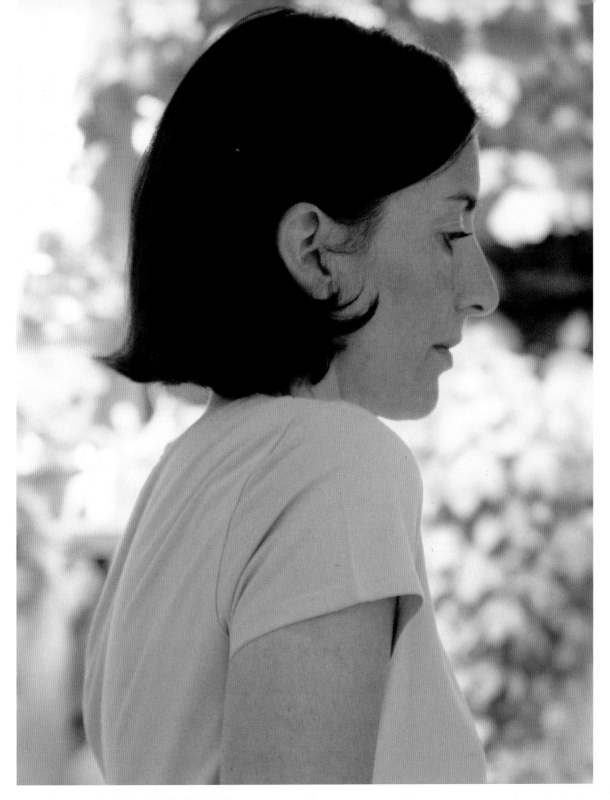

SHOULDER CIRCLES

12 **Starting in the neutral upright position,** make a circular movement with one shoulder clockwise and then anti-clockwise. Repeat with the other shoulder. Repeat up to five times on each shoulder.

FINISH by raising both shoulders up to your ears and then let them drop back down. Repeat five times.

7.Shiatsu

Shiatsu massage treatment, originating from Japan, is used to stimulate the body's natural flow of energy, helping to restore a sense of balance and wellbeing.

BACKGROUND

Shiatsu, a Japanese word that translates as "finger pressure", is a traditional therapy developed in Japan in the early twentieth century. There are a number of different styles: Zen, macrobiotic, namikoshi and hara, all of which incorporate and use theories and diagnostic techniques drawn from traditional oriental medicine. These include observation, questioning and touching, combined together with an understanding of the fundamental role of the theory of "yin and yang". Yin and yang are ways of describing apparently opposite qualities, such as hot and cold; female and male; soft and hard. In fact these qualities are complementary and necessary to each other as nothing can be wholly yin or wholly yang – one quality is meaningless without reference to the other.

This system is based on the belief that disease arises out of an imbalance between the two complementary qualities. Shiatsu aims to rectify any imbalances by working on the flow of life energy, know as "ki or chi", which circulates around the body through channels called "meridians". Ki must be kept flowing freely through the body to ensure a balance between yin and yang. There are 12 principal channels – six yin and six yang – running in pairs on either side of the body and each corresponds to an internal organ and its various functions. Shiatsu stimulates acupoints (called "tsubos"), which are located at specific points along the channels through the rhythmic application of pressure, stretching and holding techniques. This regulates the flow of ki and is thought to improve the overall function of the organs, increase the lymphatic flow, boost the circulation, release muscle tension and promote a sense of relaxation.

TECHNIQUE

A typical treatment with a professional shiatsu practitioner will take approximately an hour and will generally focus on the whole body. It is performed on a futon with the recipient wearing loose clothing, so oil or cream will not be used. The therapist will usually take a thorough case history before commencing.

You should do your shiatsu treatment on a futon or on a suitably padded floor. Both you and the person you are massaging need to wear loose, comfortable clothing.

It is better to follow the whole sequence, which will take approximately one hour.

It is vital that your posture is correct – professional therapists learn how to generate their energy from the centre of their body (the "hara") just below the naval. Try to lean your bodyweight into the person you are massaging to apply static pressure through your hands, thumbs, fingers or forearms. Your pressure should be gentle, yet firm and you will hold into the pressure techniques for up to 10 seconds. Both of your hands should remain in contact with the recipient's body throughout the treatment, with both working together, or one hand working whilst the other supports.

Try to make the techniques of palming, pressure, stretching and shaking, flow smoothly and apply them with sensitivity. Encourage the person you are treating to relax, breathe deeply and to exhale as you apply pressure.

Before you start the guided massage, you should have run through the list of contraindications on page 10–11 with the person you are going to treat. Also note that only a qualified practitioner should treat a pregnant woman. If you are both confident there is no reason why the treatment should not be given, you can begin.

The Hara is the physical centre of the body and is located just below the naval. By working from your hara, your ki or energy will flow freely through your body.

BENEFITS

Shiatsu is believed to strengthen the body's resistance to disease and relieve tension and fatigue, thus inducing relaxation.

DIAGONAL BACK STRETCH

1 **With your recipient lying on their stomach,** kneel to the right and place the palm of your right hand on the border of their left shoulder blade and your left hand on their buttocks. Lean your body weight into your arms and create a diagonal stretch between your hands. Maintain this pressure to ensure a good stretch and slowly release. Repeat once and then move to repeat it on the other side.

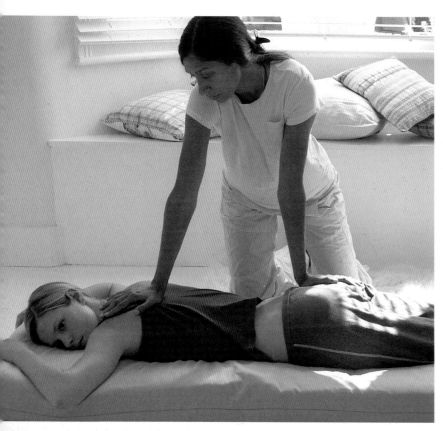

BACK PALM PRESS

2 **Place the palms of your hands between the shoulder blades on either side of the spine,** whilst kneeling on the right hand side. Lean into your arms and apply a perpendicular pressure. Maintain the pressure to ensure a good stretch and slowly release. Repeat the stretch moving down to the sacrum (the thick triangular bone situated at the base of the spine). Always try to apply the pressure when the recipient is exhaling and aim to keep your arms and back straight. Repeat.

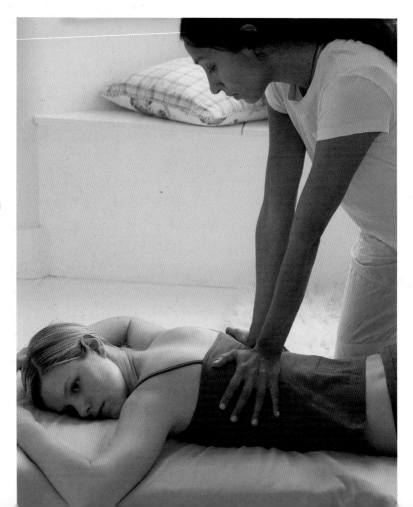

BACK PALMING

3 **Kneeling on the right side of your recipient,** place the palms of your hands between the top of the shoulders and on either side of the spine. Your fingers should be pointing toward the head and the heels of your hands towards their buttocks. Lean into your arms and alternately walk your palms down the spine to the top of the buttocks and up again. Repeat. You may feel more comfortable kneeling at the head of the recipient during this step.

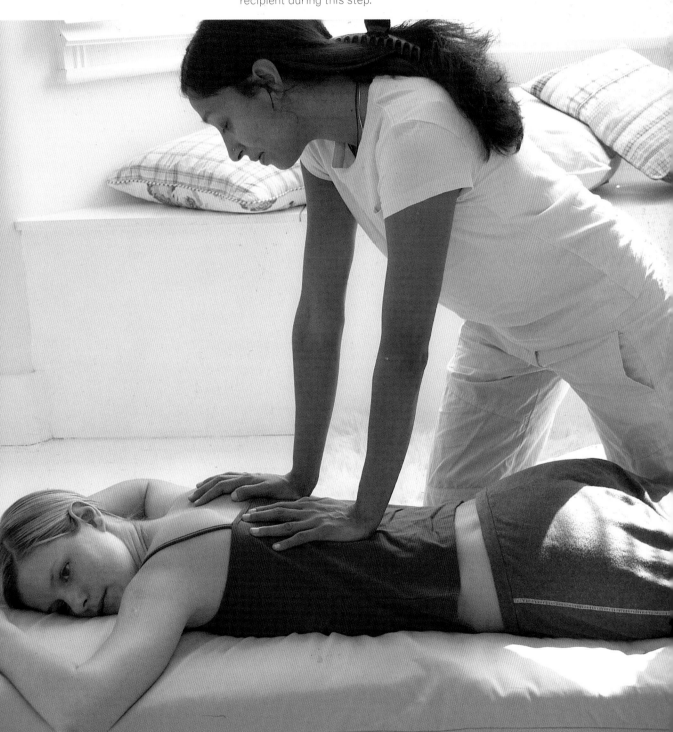

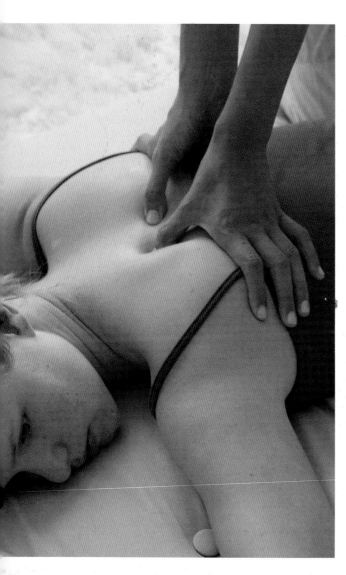

BACK THUMB PRESSURE

4 **Place your thumbs between the top of the shoulders** and on either side of the spine. Lean into your thumbs and apply a perpendicular pressure as the recipient exhales. Slowly release and work down the spine. Repeat and follow with step 3, palming.

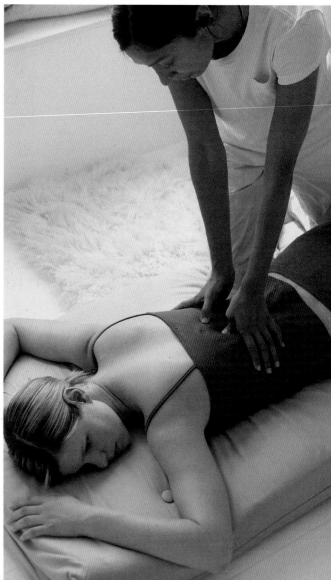

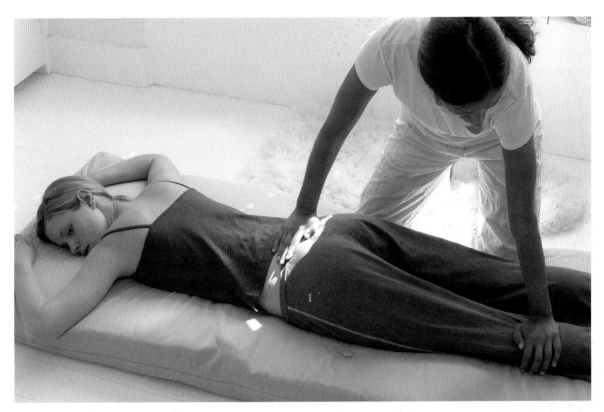

LEG PALMING

5 **Place your right arm on the sacrum and your left arm** at the top of the left thigh. The recipient's knees and toes should be pointing slightly in. You may have to adjust your posture so that you are able to palm down the leg down to the foot without overstretching or losing your balance. Lean into your arms and apply pressure down the legs with the heel of your hand. Avoid putting any pressure on the back of the knee. Repeat.

LEG STRETCH

6 **Take a hold of your recipient's ankle** and gradually bend the leg towards the buttocks. Maintain this position to ensure a good stretch and then slowly release.

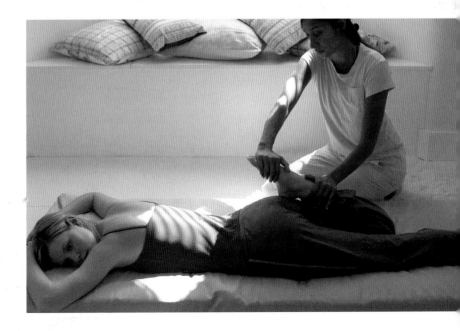

FOOT PALMING

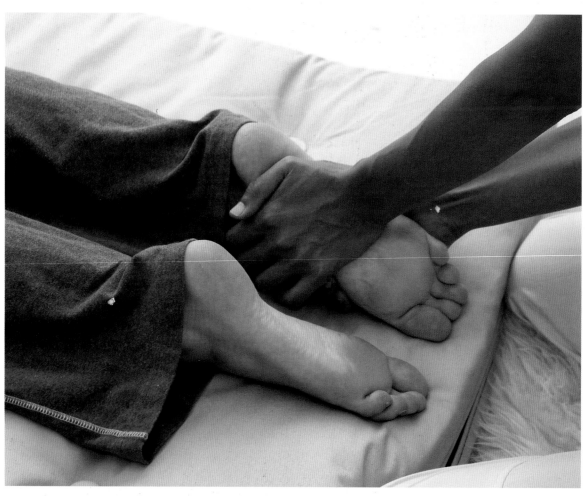

7 **Sit at the foot of the recipient** and palm the sole
of their foot with the heel of your hand.

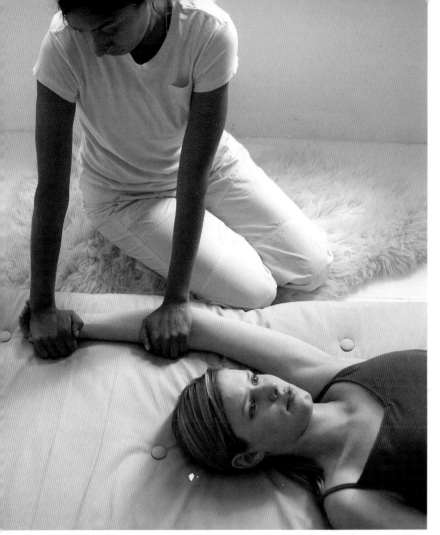

ARM STRETCH AND PALM

8 **Kneel level to the recipient's head** and, holding the arm at the wrist and inside the elbow, rotate the arm into an overhead stretch. Release the stretch, move the arm back onto the futon (or floor) and palm from the wrist to the underarm.

HAND STRETCH

9 **Rotate your body so that you are facing** your recipient's hand. Cup the back of the hand in your fingers and stretch the palm open with your thumbs. Repeat and return the arm to the recipient's side.

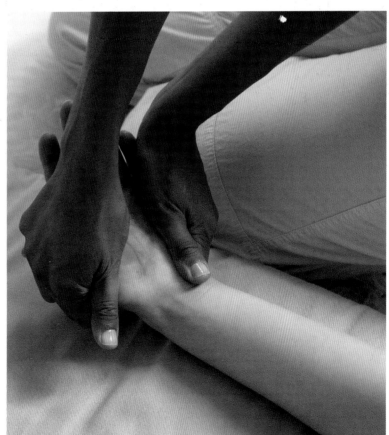

SQUEEZE AND STRETCH THE FINGERS

10 **Return to the side of your recipient** and, holding the hand, squeeze up the fleshy areas of the arm from wrist to shoulder. Holding the wrist, lift the arm off the floor and gently shake it out. Repeat this until the arm feels relaxed and floppy. Now squeeze every finger between your thumb and forefinger from the knuckle to the fingertip.

Repeat steps 9–11 on the other arm.

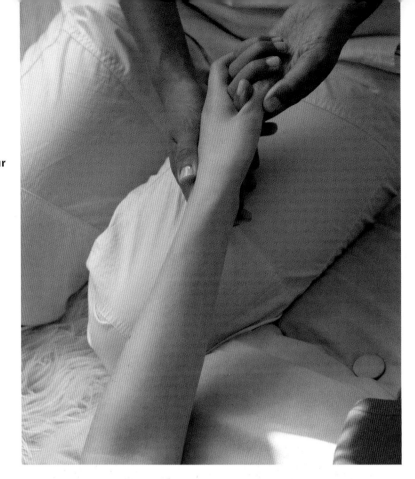

SHOULDER SQUEEZING

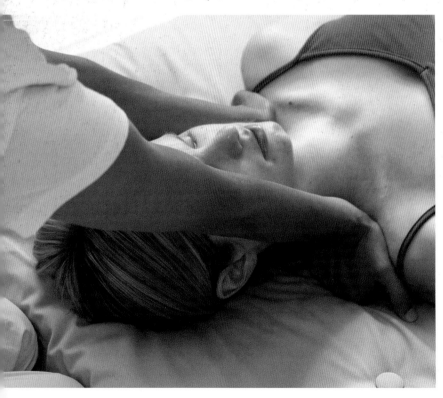

11 **Kneel at the head of your recipient** and place the palms of your hands on the shoulders. Your fingers should be pointing down the arms. As they exhale, apply a downward pressure through your straight arms. This move will stretch and open the chest. Hold the stretch for up to 30 seconds and release. Repeat a couple of times. Place your fingers under the shoulders and palm the shoulders between the heel of your hands and your fingers.

NECK SQUEEZING

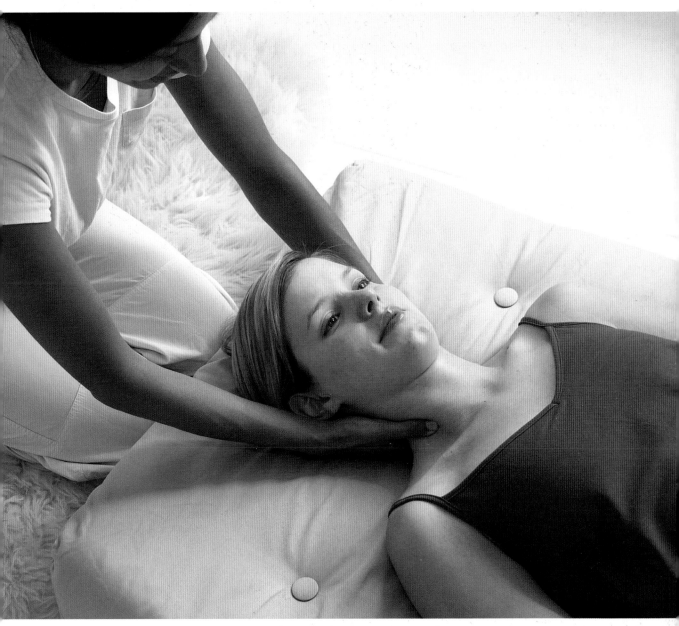

12 **Kneeling at the head of the recipient,** with your fingers underneath the neck and your thumbs on either side, squeeze the neck muscles between the heel of your hand and your fingers. Work up the neck to the base of the skull and repeat back down. Cradle the neck in your fingers and gently pull your hands upwards and away. Repeat this stretch until you feel the neck relax.

Finish the shiatsu session by resting the recipient's head in your hands for 30 seconds.

> **THE PERSON** you have massaged will probably need at least a few minutes before they feel ready to get up. Help them to get up if necessary and advise them to drink plenty of water.

8. Acupressure

Acupressure is the application of pressure using the fingertips or thumbs on specific points on the body – known as acupoints – to alleviate pain, relieve muscle tension and stimulate the internal organs.

BACKGROUND

Acupressure is another method that dates back thousands of years. It was traditionally used as a form of first-aid treatment and self-care regime in ancient China and Japan. It is often described as "acupuncture without the needles" ("acus" is the Latin word for needles). The Chinese believed that pressing certain points on the body relieved pain and also gave overall health benefits throughout the body. Acupressure not only alleviates pain, but can also help to relieve muscle tension, stimulate the internal organs, and have a positive effect on heart rate, blood pressure and circulation.

Like shiatsu, acupressure is based on the beliefs of traditional Chinese medicine and the theory of yin and yang. Acupressure is the application of pressure with the fingertip or thumb on the acupoints located along the body's 12 channels or "meridians". It is believed there are over 360 bilateral acupoints in the body, each one relating to a specific organ or body system. They are numbered and named according to the meridian on which they lie. The points below the elbows and knees are generally thought to be more effective than those above. Again, as with shiatsu, the principle of the treatment is to balance and ensure the proper flow of ki energy. A free flow of ki helps to maintain good health, while depleted ki can lead to illness.

TECHNIQUE

These guided acupressure self-help treatments require no equipment. You could do them seated or lying down, and you do not need any oil or cream. Follow the guided instructions to locate your acupoint. Acupoints tend to sit in small depressions between bones, muscles or tendons and they will feel mildly tender to the touch.

Once you have located the point, gently stimulate or rub it with your fingertip or thumb, increasing the pressure gradually – you may feel a slight sensation but your treatment should never result in pain. Apply the pressure for no more than two minutes and if the point is very sensitive, move to the diametrically opposing or alternatively related point. You should always treat both sides of the body except when working on the spine or midline of the body.

For acute conditions, self-treatment can be applied at hourly intervals. Decrease frequency as your condition improves. Applying acupressure little and often is much more beneficial than longer periods at irregular intervals. For non-acute conditions, treatment two to three times a week is usually sufficient.

Before you start the guided massage, consider whether any of the contraindications on pages 10–11 apply to you. Note that although areas of inflammation, swelling, open wounds or sores cannot be treated directly, pressure may be applied to the next nearest point. Do not apply the techniques if you are pregnant. If you are confident that there is no reason not to do these techniques, you can begin.

Gently stimulate or rub an acupoint with your fingertips or thumbs, increasing the pressure gradually – the treatment should never be painful.

BENEFITS

Acupressure may be used to prevent or ease minor common ailments, such as headaches, eye strain, sinus problems, toothache, menstrual cramps, constipation, indigestion, muscle aches, stress and lower backache. It is believed to positively influence the functioning of the internal organs.

NAUSEA/TRAVEL SICKNESS

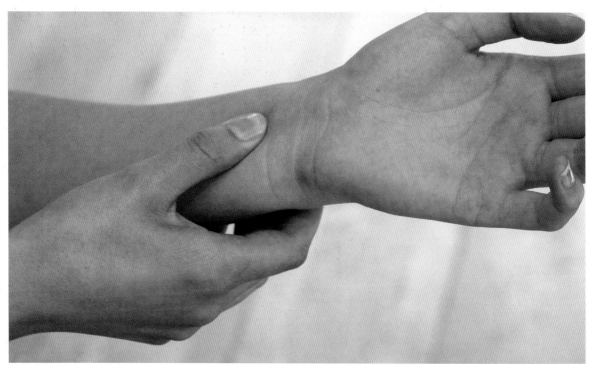

1 **Rest one of your wrists in the palm of your other hand** and
apply pressure with the thumb to pericardium 6. To locate this point,
measure two-and-a-half fingers' width from the wrist crease up inside
your forearm and place your thumb between the tendons. Slowly apply
pressure and gently stimulate the point for up to one minute, before
releasing. Repeat on the other arm.

HEADACHES, NECK AND SHOULDER ACHE

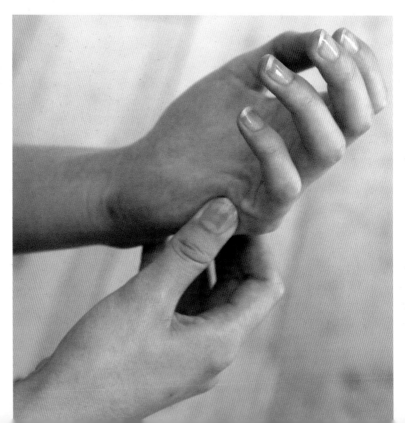

2 **Rest one hand in the palm
of your other hand** and apply
pressure with the thumb to small
intestine 3. To locate this point,
make a loose fist with your hand
and place your thumb on the
longest crease on the outside
edge of your little finger. Slowly
apply pressure and gently
stimulate the point for up to
one minute, before releasing.
Repeat on the other hand.

AGITATION, DIZZINESS AND TEMPERATURE

3 **Applying pressure with the thumb or forefinger** to lung 11 can reduce agitation, dizziness and a high temperature. Lung 11 is located on the outside edge of the thumb by the corner of the nail. Slowly apply pressure and gently stimulate the point for up to one minute, before releasing. Repeat on the other hand.

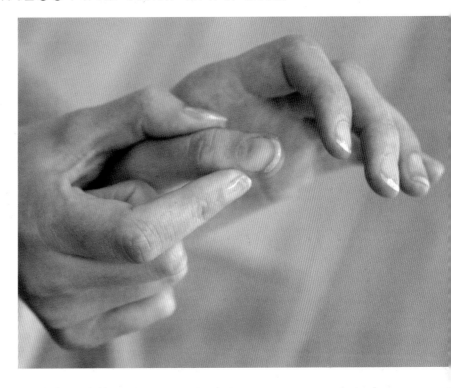

THE COMMON COLD

4 **Rest one hand on the fingers of your other hand** and apply pressure with the thumb to large intestine 4 to alleviate the symptoms of the common cold. Large intestine 4 is located on the back of the hand, in the centre of the triangle created between the bones of the thumb and forefinger. Slowly apply pressure and gently stimulate the point for up to one minute, before releasing. Repeat on the other hand.

INSOMNIA

5 **Supporting one wrist with the other hand,** apply pressure with the thumb or forefinger to heart 7, to alleviate insomnia. Heart 7 is located on the palm side of the hand a quarter way along the wrist crease, in alignment with the little finger.

Slowly apply pressure and gently stimulate the point for up to one minute, before releasing. Repeat on the other wrist.

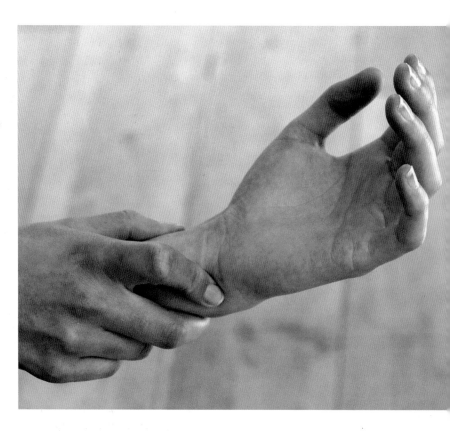

PERIOD PAIN AND HANGOVER

6 **To relieve period pain and hangovers,** apply pressure with your thumb to liver 3. Liver 3 is located on top of the foot, two thumbs' width above the web, in the depression between the first and second toes. Slowly apply pressure and gently stimulate the point for up to one minute, before releasing. Repeat on the other foot.

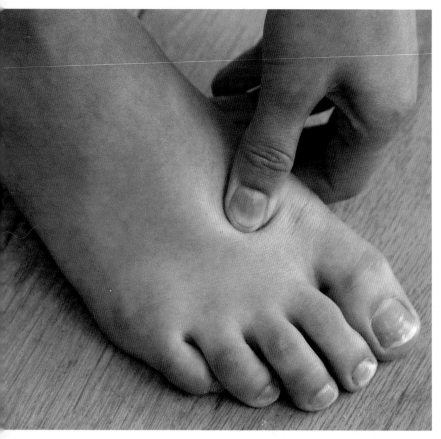

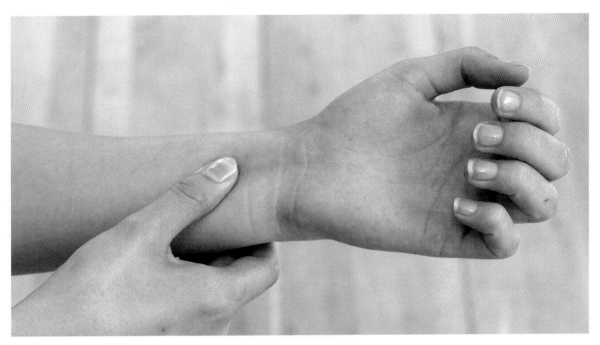

ANXIETY

7 **Rest one wrist in the palm of your other hand** and apply pressure with your thumb to pericardium 6. To locate this point, measure two-and-a-half fingers' width from the wrist crease up inside your forearm and place your thumb between the tendons. Slowly apply pressure and gently stimulate the point for up to one minute, before releasing. Repeat on the other wrist.

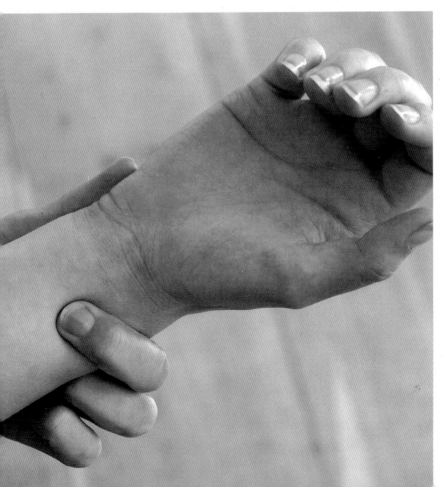

SORE THROAT

8 **Rest one wrist in the palm of your other hand** and apply pressure with your thumb or forefinger to lung 7. Lung 7 is located palm up and two fingers above the wrist crease, in line with the thumb. Slowly apply pressure and gently stimulate the point for up to one minute, before releasing. Repeat on the other wrist.

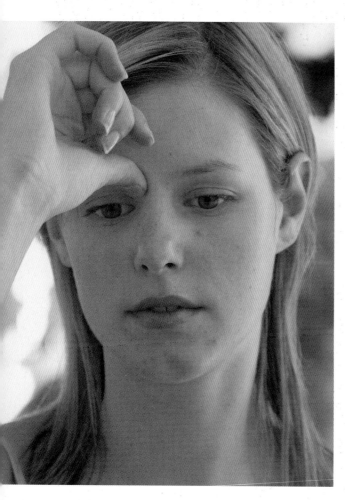

BLOCKED SINUSES

9 **Applying pressure with your thumb** to bladder 2 will help to clear the sinuses. Bladder 2 is located on the inner edge of the eyebrow. Slowly apply pressure and gently stimulate the point for up to one minute, before releasing. Repeat on the other side.

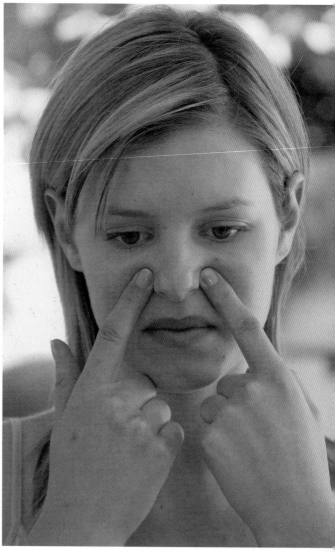

NOSEBLEEDS

10 **To help stop or prevent a nosebleed,** apply pressure with your thumbs to the point directly below the pupil on either side of the nostrils at the base of the nose. Slowly apply pressure and gently stimulate the point for up to one minute, before releasing. Repeat if necessary. This point is not named on a meridian.

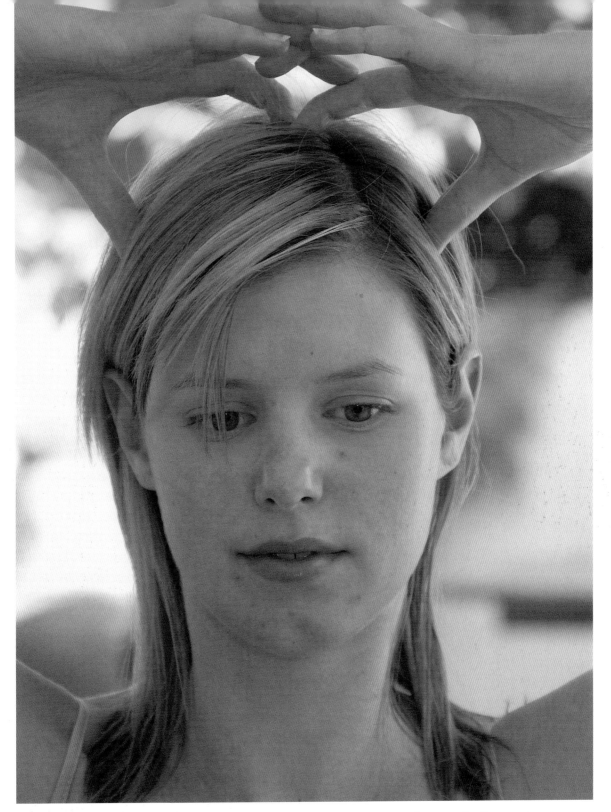

MEMORY AND CONCENTRATION

11 **To improve your memory and concentration,** apply pressure with your forefingers to governor vessel 20. Governor vessel 20 is located on top of the head, in line with the nose. Slowly apply pressure and gently stimulate the point for up to one minute, before releasing. Repeat.

SQUEEZING THE SHOULDERS

1 **Standing behind your seated recipient,** gently squeeze the large muscles on either side of the upper back (the trapezius) between the fingers and heels of both hands. With one hand on either side of the back, use alternating pressure to cover most of the shoulder area. Repeat a couple of times.

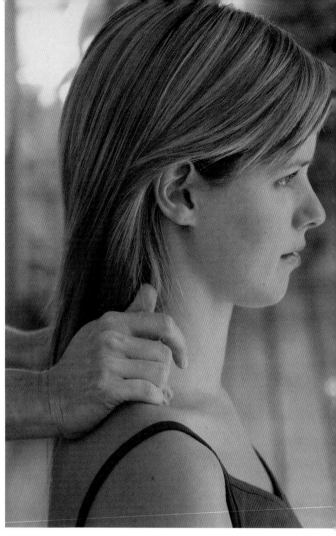

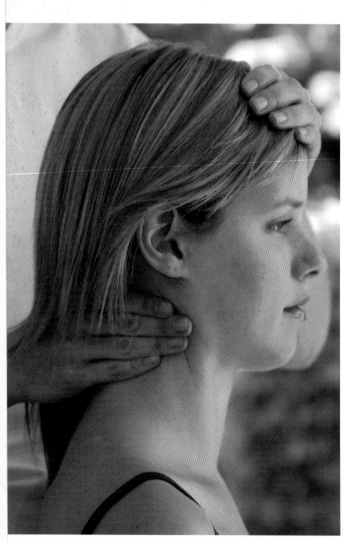

KNEADING THE NECK

2 **Stand to the left of your recipient.** Supporting the head with your left hand, with your right hand, squeeze up the neck and around the base of the skull with gentle kneading and stretching movements. Repeat a couple of times.

THUMB
PRESSURE AT
BASE OF SKULL

3 **Stand in the same position as step 2** and, still supporting the recipient's head, apply small circular pressures up around the base of the skull. Start in the centre of the neck and work out towards the ears. Repeat a couple of times.

Repeat steps 2 and 3 on the right-hand side of the neck.

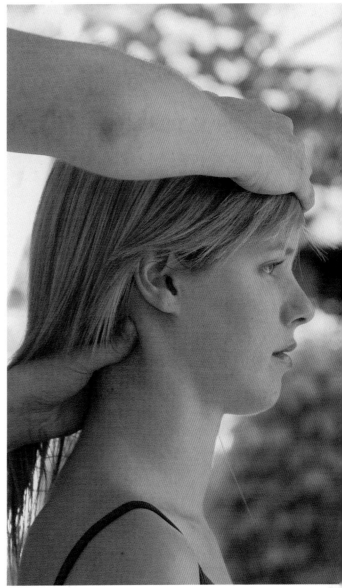

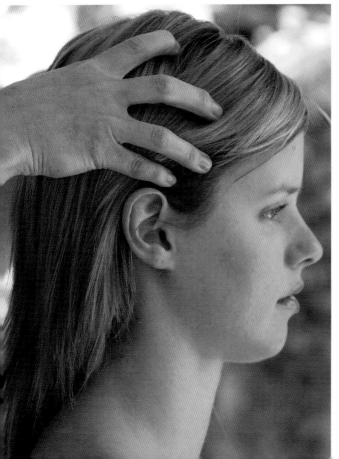

SCALP MASSAGE

4 **Standing directly behind the recipient,** massage the scalp with your fingertips in firm circular movements as though washing the hair. Feel for areas of tension where the muscles hardly move and try to move the skin over the scalp, without letting your fingers slip through the hair. Do extra work in the hollows at the base of the skull and pay attention lo areas of tension. Make the movements slow and rhythmical, repeating them until you feel the tightness loosening.

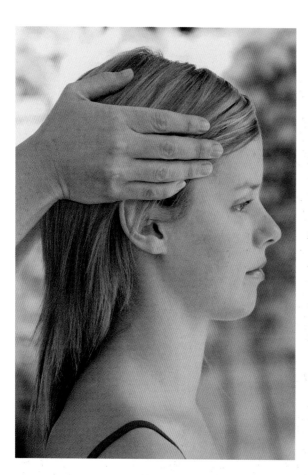

SQUEEZING
THE SCALP

5 **Standing directly behind the recipient,** place the palms of both your hands around their scalp like a cap. Now squeeze, lift slightly and release. Repeat several times. This movement is very soothing and can be used as a self-help technique to cure headaches.

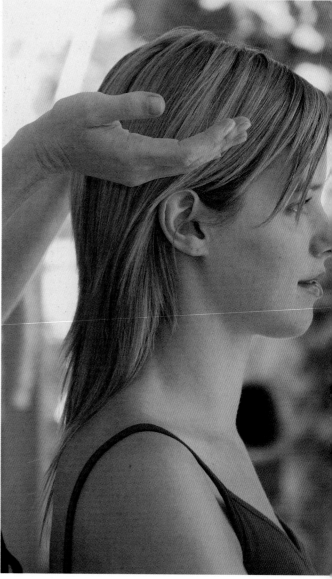

COMBING THROUGH THE HAIR

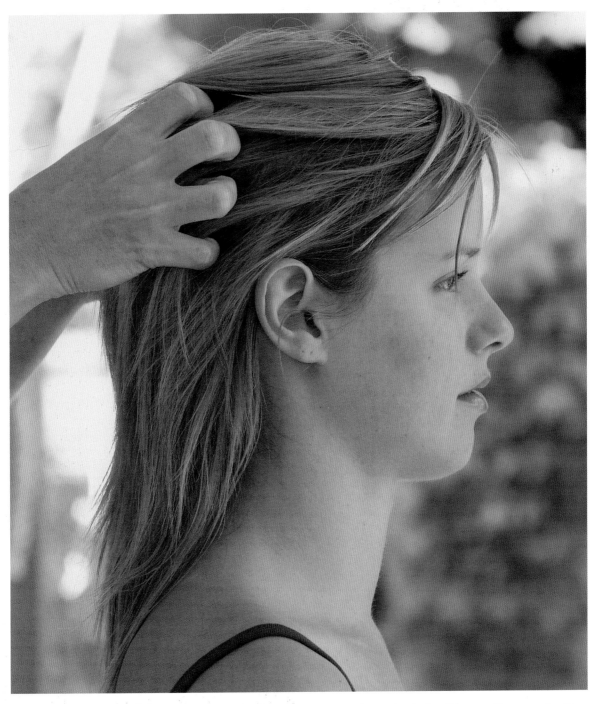

6 **Calm the scalp by combing the hair with your fingers** – it will give the feeling that tension is gently being lifted out of the scalp. Start by combing the hair at the hairline, gradually working towards the crown of the head and through to the ends. Repeat several times.

FOREHEAD LIFT

7 **This is similar to step 5,** but this time you place the palms of your hands on the recipient's temples and your fingers on the forehead. Squeeze, lift slightly and release. It is great for drawing stress out of the face. Repeat several times.

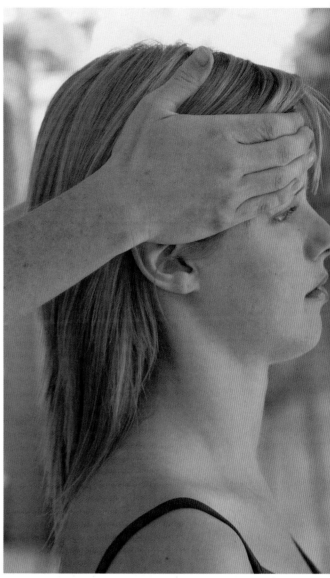

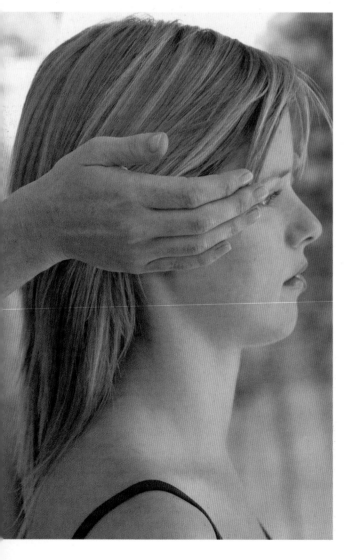

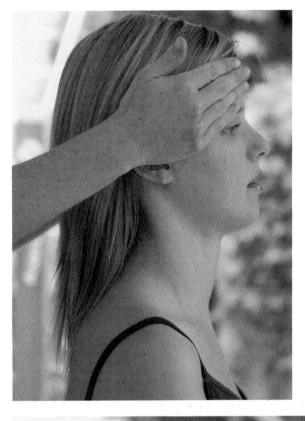

FACE MASSAGE

8 **Place the palms of your hands on the temples** and your fingers on the forehead to stroke the face very lightly. Starting from the forehead, work down the face to the chin. Gently flick your hands away from the chin, return to the forehead and repeat. This is a good self-help exercise to treat insomnia.

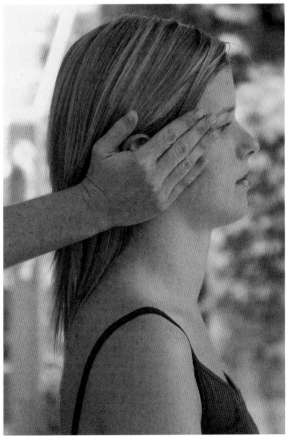

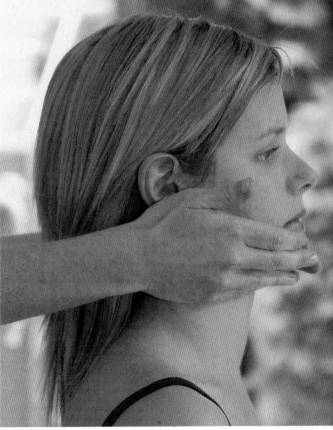

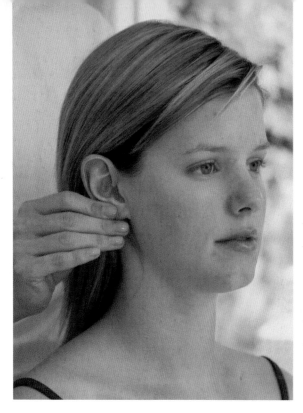

EAR MASSAGE

9 Massage around the ears and in the ear margin. Now gently squeeze the flesh, working down to the ear lobes. Massaging the ears is highly beneficial, as they contain a number of acupressure points relating to different areas of the body.

BRUSHING DOWN THE BACK

10 Place your hands on the top of the recipient's shoulders and brush them down the back. Return your hand to the shoulders and brush them down the arms. Repeat several times. These movements should not be too fast or slow. Try to mould your hands along the surface of the body.

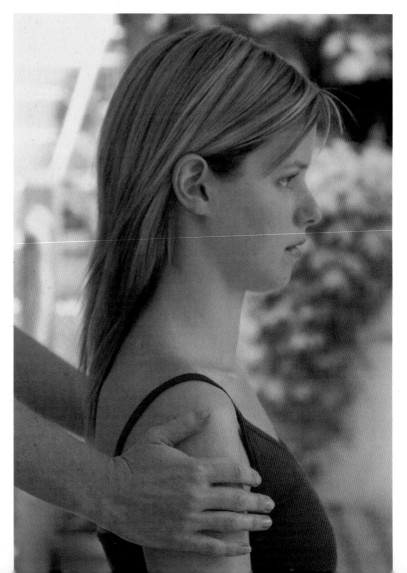

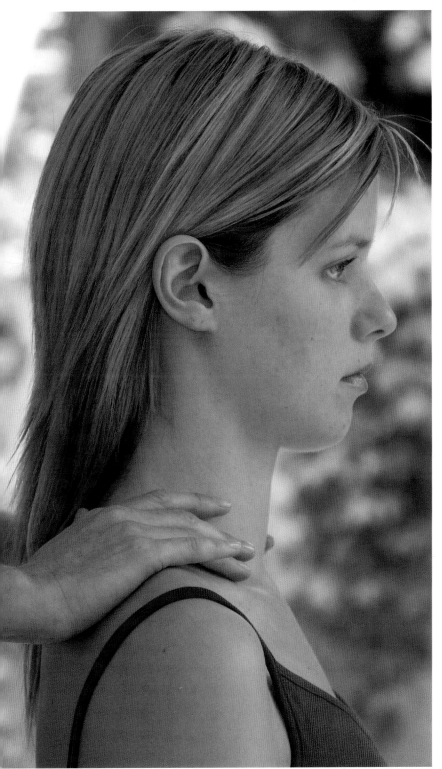

FINISHING

11 **Place your hands on the recipient's shoulders** and hold for up to 30 seconds, while you both relax and focus on your breathing. This allows the recipient a final short period of calmness before the end of the treatment.

THE PERSON you have massaged will probably need at least a few minutes before they feel ready to get up. Help them to get up if necessary and advise them to drink plenty of water.

10. On-site/seated massage

On-site massage is a form of bodywork that can be done almost anywhere and is ideal for the needs of the workspace. It can help to improve office energy and morale, thus increasing productivity and reducing absenteeism.

BACKGROUND

On-site massage was developed in the early 1980s by an American practitioner called David Palmer. He recognized a market for massage in the workplace and developed a system that was both portable and convenient. On-site massage has since become hugely popular and common in many offices, convention halls, airports, studios and call centres. In fact the treatment can be given almost anywhere and many people who would not normally consider having a massage feel confident about trying it.

It combines a traditional approach to massage with the contemporary demands of busy working schedules to give the maximum effect within a limited time. On-site massage incorporates both Swedish and shiatsu-style techniques to access the soft tissue and meridians of the back, neck, shoulders, arms and hands.

The method incorporates a set sequence called a "kata" and it follows the theory of yin and yang, aiming to balance the flow of ki through the body's meridians. As with acupressure, on-site massage aims to rectify any imbalances by stimulating the acupoints through pressure, stretching and holding techniques. It is believed that applying pressure to these points will enhance the flow of ki and hence alleviate tension and anxiety.

TECHNIQUE

A typical on-site massage session takes 15 to 20 minutes and does not require the removal of clothes or the use of oil. The therapist doesn't need to take a case history, but may ask some basic screening questions. The client usually sits in a specially designed chair (an ergonomic chair), which supports the shoulders, back, neck, arms, hands and head while the massage takes place.

However, it's very easy to do this treatment using an ordinary chair. An on-site massage kata is tightly choreographed, so follow all the guided steps, which will take approximately 20 minutes. Try to keep your sequence as smooth and flowing as possible, applying all the techniques with sensitivity and paying extra attention to areas of tension.

The techniques include kneading, palming, squeezing, pressure and tapotement. Try to lean your bodyweight into the person you are massaging to apply static pressure through your hands, thumbs, fingers or forearms. Both of your hands will be in contact with the recipient's body throughout the treatment, with both working together or one hand working whilst the other supports.

On-site massage incorporates both Swedish and Shiatsu-style techniques to access the soft tissue and meridians of the back, neck, shoulders, arms and hands.

Ask the person you are going to treat where they are feeling most tense or whether they are suffering from a headache or eye strain (common conditions for people who spend long periods in front of a computer or machinery).

Before you start the guided massage, you should have run through the list of contraindications on pages 10–11 with the person you are going to treat. If you are both confident that there is no reason why the treatment should not be given, you can begin.

BENEFITS

On-site massage has been found to provide quick, effective stress release and relaxation. It may enhance productivity in a working environment, by increasing energy and concentration, and improving office morale.

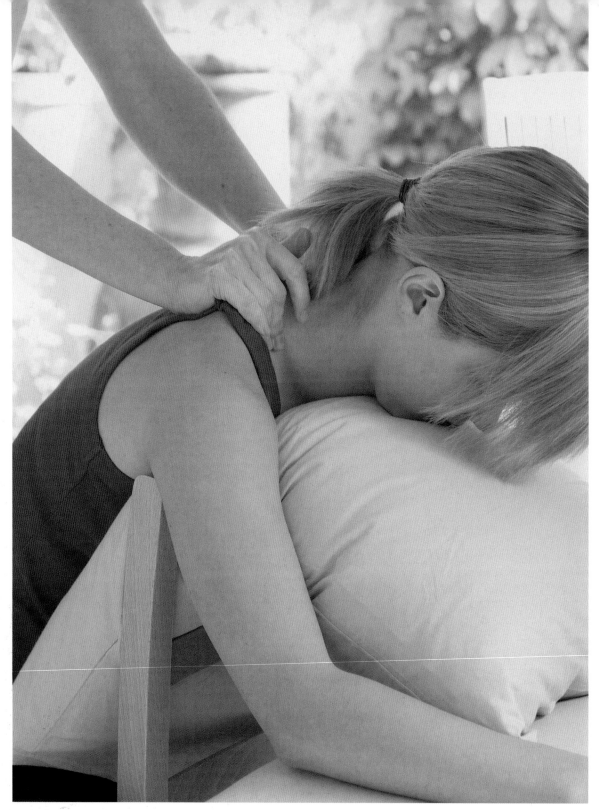

KNEADING THE SHOULDERS

1 **Place a pillow over the back of a standard kitchen chair.** Ask your recipient to sit astride it and lean forwards into the pillow. Stand behind the chair and place your hands on the shoulders and knead the shoulders either together or alternately. Make sure you cover the whole shoulder area. Repeat several times.

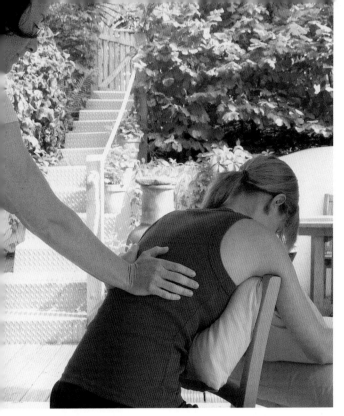

DOUBLE PALM PRESS

2 **Place the heels of your hands on either side** of the spine with your fingers pointing out to the ribs. Starting just below the shoulder blade, lean your body weight through straight arms to apply pressure through five points down the back to the sacrum. Both you and the recipient should exhale on each press. Repeat.

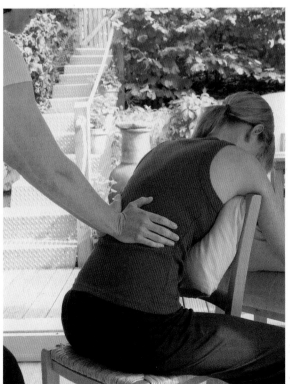

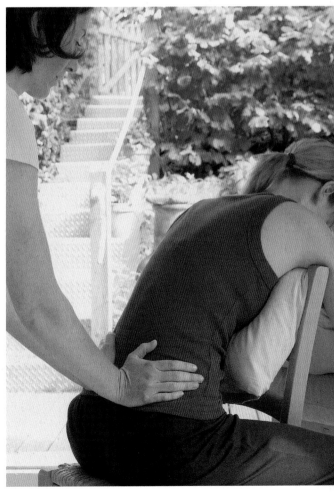

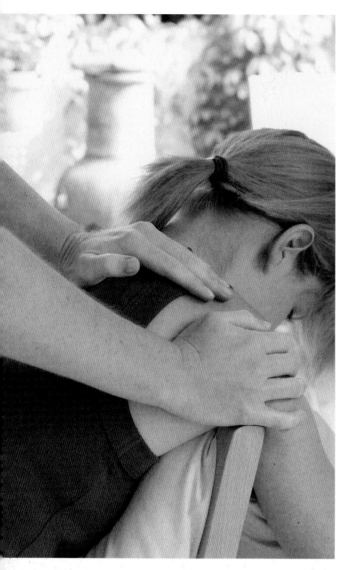

PALM PRESS AROUND THE SHOULDER BLADE

3 **Press the heel of your right hand** around the outline of the shoulder blade and lean your body weight forward to apply a downward and outward pressure. Your other hand should rest on and support the recipient's shoulder. There should be very little motion in this stretch. Repeat.

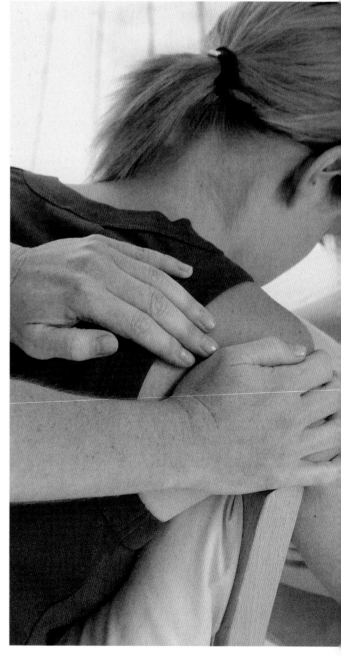

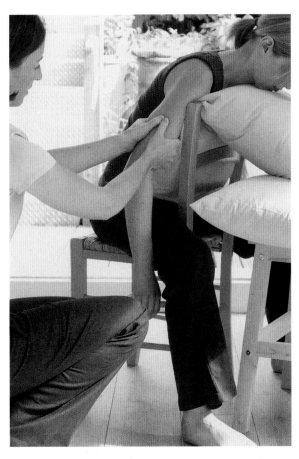

ARM MASSAGE

4 **Kneel at the side of your recipient** facing their arm. Try not to bend your back as you squeeze the arm between your palms and fingers, from the top to the wrist. Return to the top of the arm and apply pressure with your thumbs to five evenly spaced points down the centre of the arm to end just above the elbow. Repeat.

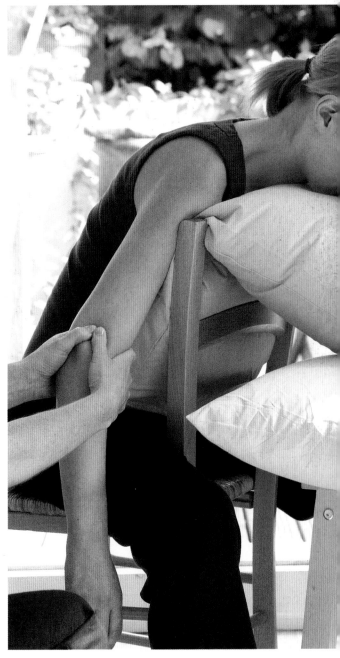

FOREARM
MASSAGE

5 **Kneel at the side of your recipient** facing the arm. Support the wrist with one hand whilst applying pressure with the thumb of your free hand to five evenly spaced points down the centre of the forearm from just below the elbow to the wrist crease. Repeat.

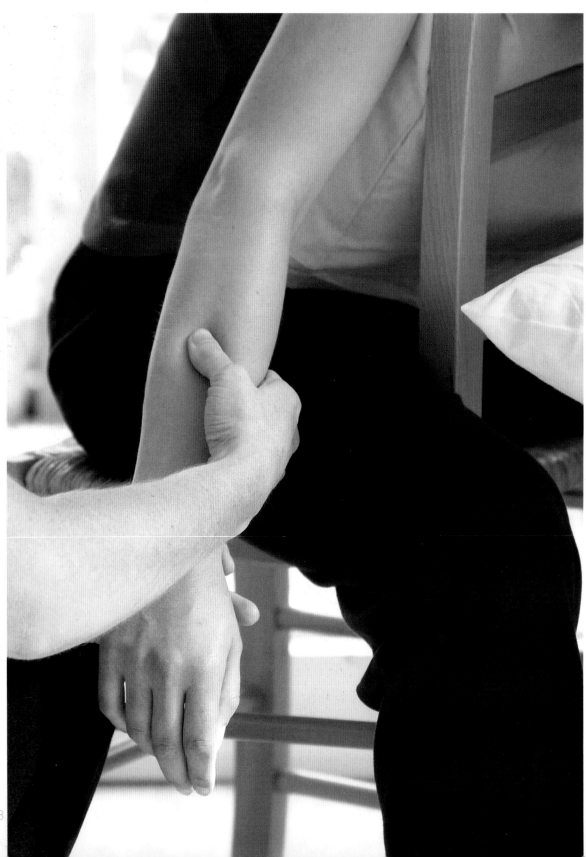

HAND MASSAGE

6 **Move to the front of your recipient** and, supporting the wrist with one hand, rotate the forearm so that you can squeeze the fleshy area of the inner arm from the elbow to the thumb side of the wrist. Repeat.

Grasp the hand (with your fingers underneath and your thumbs together in the centre of the palm) and stretch out the hand by pulling your thumbs out towards the edges of the palm. Repeat. Release the arm back to the side.

Repeat steps 3–6 on the other arm and hand.

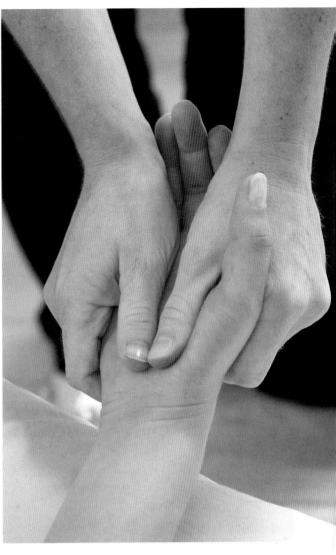

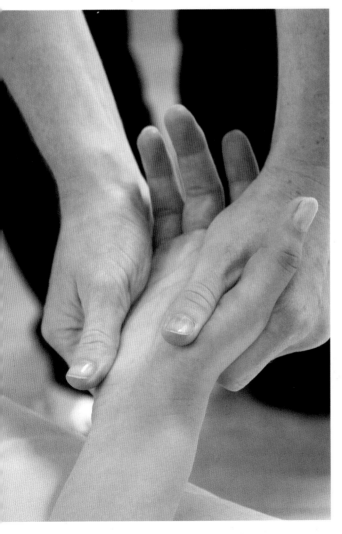

LOWER BACK
PALM PRESS

7 **Standing behind the recipient,** repeat step 2, double palm press. Now place one of your hands on the shoulder and the heel of your other hand next to the spine on the opposite side. Starting below the ribs lean your bodyweight forward to apply pressure down three points to the sacrum. Remember to exhale as you apply pressure. Repeat.

Repeat on the other shoulder.

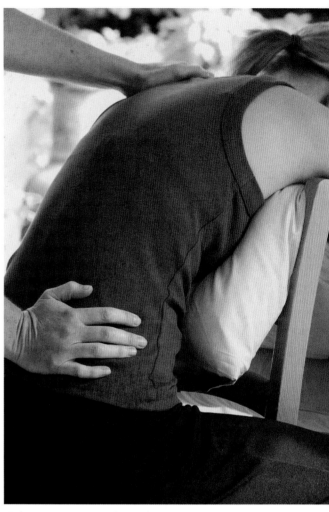

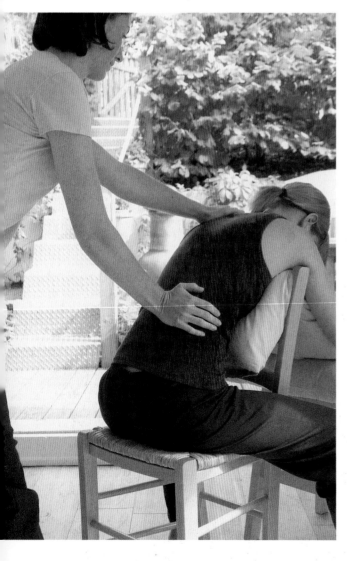

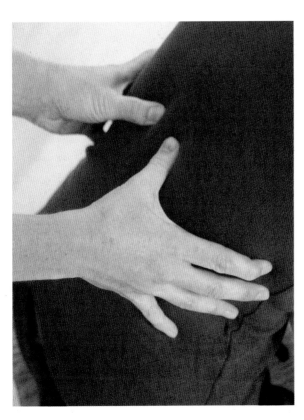

THUMB PRESSURE DOWN THE SPINE

8 Standing directly behind the recipient, lean your body-weight into your thumbs and apply pressure to nine points down either side of the spine. Start below the shoulder blade and work at evenly spaced points down to the sacrum. Repeat and follow with step 2, double palm press.

NECK MASSAGE

9 Move to the right of the recipient. Support the head with your right hand as your left hand gently squeezes up the neck and around the base of the skull. Repeat once and then work from the left-hand side.

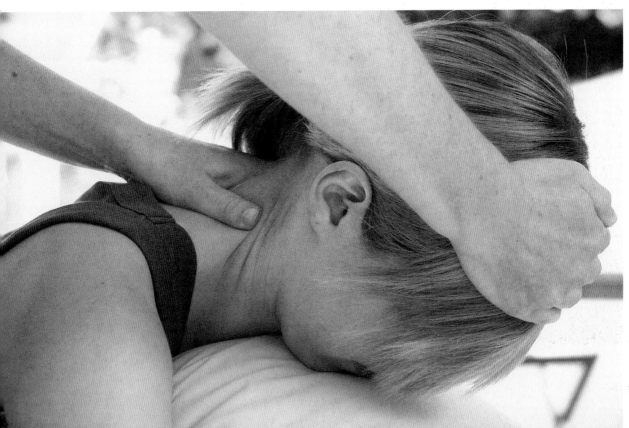

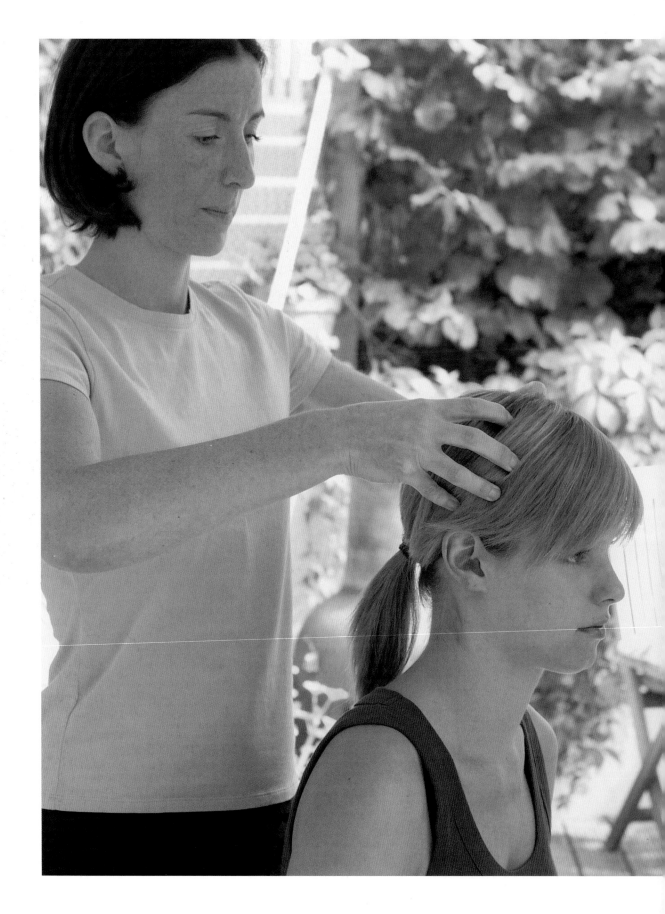

SCALP
MASSAGE

10 Ask your recipient to sit upright, but keep a gentle hold on the shoulders until they are stabilized – some people may feel dizzy. Massage the scalp with your fingertips in firm circular movements as though washing the hair. Feel for areas of tension where the scalp is tight and try to move the skin over the scalp without letting your fingers slip through the hair. Make the movements slow and rhythmical. Repeat until you feel the scalp loosening under your fingers.

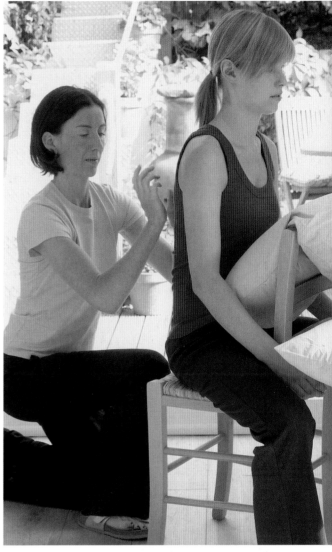

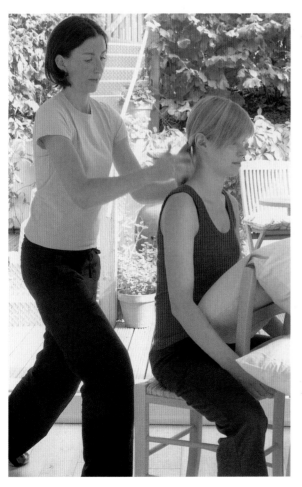

PERCUSSION

11 With loose wrists and relaxed fingers, apply quick hacking strokes with alternate hands, across the shoulders and up and down either side of the spine. Be careful over the lower back area. Repeat. Lightly brush your hands down the arms and back before resting them on the recipient's shoulders for 30 seconds.

THE PERSON you have massaged will probably need at least a few minutes before they feel ready to get up. Help them to get up if necessary and advise them to drink plenty of water.

11. Tui Na

Tui Na is a deep and vigorous treatment used to treat internal imbalances, musculo-skeletal ailments and to enhance the body's resistance to disease.

BACKGROUND

Tui Na dates back thousands of years to the time of the ancient Chinese Shang dynasty, but is still in use today in hospitals around China. The name Tui Na comes from the root words "tui" (to push) and "na" (to lift and squeeze). It is believed that shiatsu was created when Tui Na was introduced to Japan over 1000 years ago. Tui Na is another therapy that uses the beliefs of traditional Chinese medicine and the theory of yin and yang, believing that disease arises out of an imbalance between these two elements. Both systems are used to treat internal imbalances, musculo-skeletal ailments and to enhance the body's resistance to disease. Shiatsu, however, applies slow and sustained techniques whilst Tui Na is a deep and vigorous treatment.

Tui Na focuses on the same 12 channels and acupoints of the body as shiatsu. Ki energy flows through these channels and may be affected by many physical or emotional issues.

As well as treating muscles and joints, Tui Na seeks to ensure the proper flow of this ki energy to maintain the body in a state of good health. It uses a variety of movements to manipulate the meridians and acupoints to treat localized problems and more general conditions. Both sides of the body should be treated in unison unless you are working on the midline of the body or you are treating a specific pain – in this instance, only the injured side need be treated.

TECHNIQUE

A professional Tui Na treatment can last from 30 to 90 minutes. It is given through loose clothing and does not involve the use of oil. The therapist will usually take a full case history. Many therapists will start a treatment with the client sitting, so that they can work on the neck, shoulders, arms and hands. Then the client lies down for treatment of the back, legs, feet, the face, head and neck.

The techniques used in Tui Na involve vigorous and penetrating pulling, pushing, plucking, squeezing, kneading and rolling of the soft tissues of the body, combined with manipulation of joints to regulate the flow of ki. The techniques are applied with the fingers, thumb, elbow, knuckles and the heel of the hand. Advanced therapists may also use herbal poultices, compresses, liniments and salves to enhance the therapeutic effect of the treatment.

You can give a Tui Na treatment on a massage couch, a futon or on a suitably padded floor. Both you and the person you are massaging should wear loose, comfortable clothing. Following the whole sequence will take approximately an hour.

Try to make your sequence flow smoothly and apply the techniques with sensitivity.

You will use rocking, pressing, kneading, thumb plucks, rolling, stretching and tapotement techniques in the guided massage. Try to lean your bodyweight into the person you are massaging to apply pressure through your hands, thumbs or fingers. Both of your hands will be in contact with the recipient's body throughout the treatment, with both hands working together or one hand working whilst the other supports.

Tui Na focuses on the same 12 channels and acupoints of the body as Shiatsu. Ki energy flows through these channels and may be affected by many physical or emotional issues.

Pressure should be deep and firm, but apply it gradually. Always get feedback to ensure the person you are treating is not feeling any discomfort. Encourage them to relax, breathe deeply and to exhale as you apply pressure.

Before you start the guided massage, you should have run through the list of contraindications on pages 10–11 with the person you are going to treat. Note that only a professional therapist should treat a pregnant woman. If you are both confident that there is no reason why the treatment should not be given, you can begin.

BENEFITS

Tui Na can reduce and relieve stress, promoting vitality. It is believed to boost the immune system, help heal injury and realign the musculo-skeletal system.

ROCKING
THE HIPS

1 **With the recipient lying on their stomach,** stand to the right and place your hands flat across the sacrum. Now gently push the hips from side to side in a rocking motion. Continue for a few minutes.

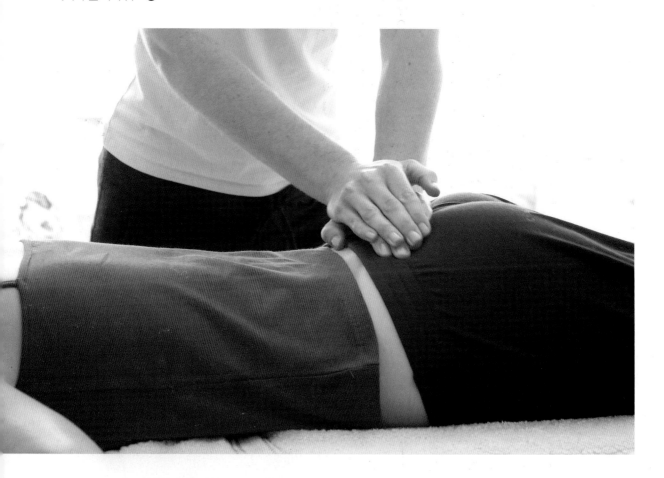

APPLYING PRESSURE

2 **Continue rocking as you move your right hand** from the sacrum and place it under the left shoulder blade. Your fingers should be facing away from you and the heel of your hand should be resting against the spine. Now apply pressure through your right hand and push the spinal muscles away from the spine. Continue down the back from the shoulder blade to the sacrum. Repeat several times. Repeat on the right-hand side of the body. Always begin with gentle pressure, increasing and decreasing it gradually.

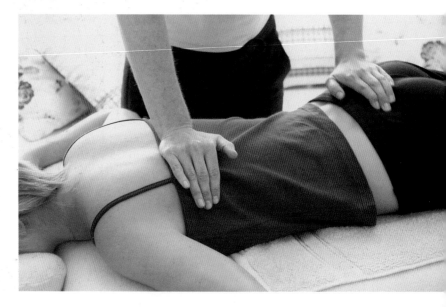

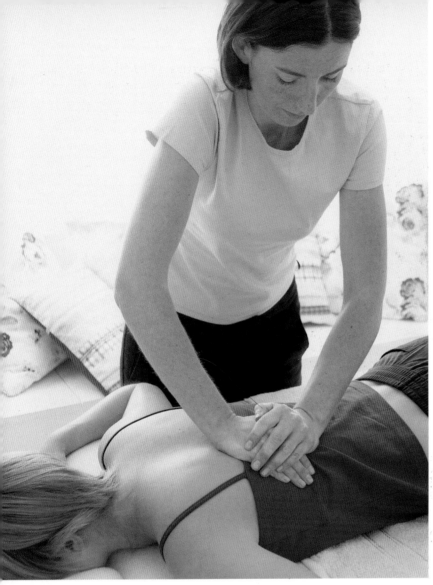

KNEADING THE SPINAL MUSCLES

3 **With one hand on top of the other** and the fingers of your left hand crossing the fingers of your right hand, knead the spinal muscles in a circular motion with the heels of your hands. Start between the left shoulder blades and gradually move down the back to the sacrum, trying to relax the spinal muscles. Repeat on the right-hand side. Always begin with gentle pressure, increasing and decreasing it gradually.

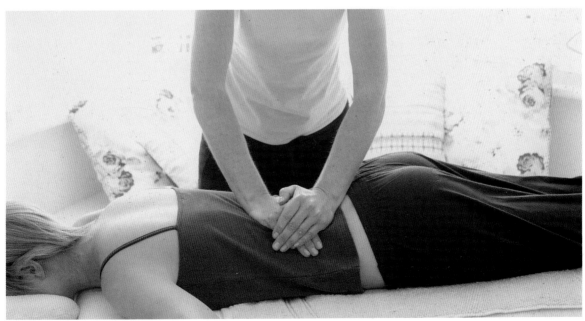

USING THE HEEL
OF YOUR HAND

4 **Place the heel of your left hand on the left-hand edge of the spine** and support your arm with your right hand. Apply pressure through the heel of your left hand and slowly push away from you and over the spinal muscles. Now pull the heel of your hand back over the muscle. Continue this rocking motion backwards and forwards, trying to get the muscles to relax. Move down the spine to the sacrum. Repeat from the right-hand edge of the spinal muscles down the body.

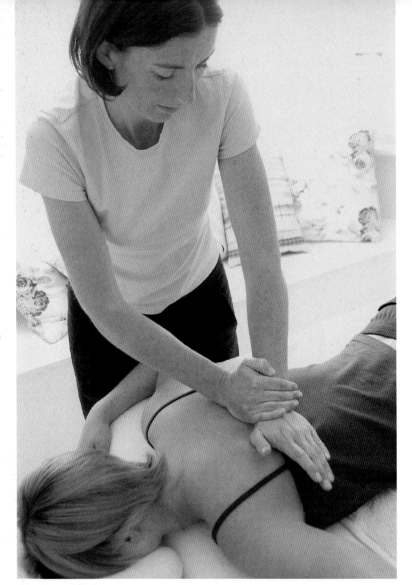

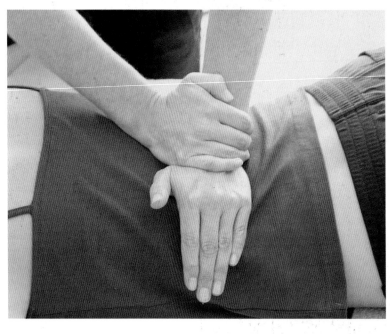

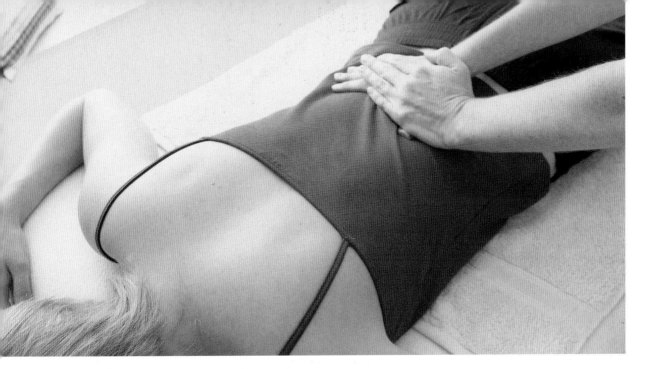

THUMB PLUCKING

5 **Standing or kneeling on the left side of the recipient,** place the pad of your right thumb on the left spinal muscle. Place the heel of your left hand on top of your thumb and apply pressure through the thumb. Push forwards over the spinal muscles towards the spine and then pull backwards. Repeat this plucking and rocking action, trying to relax the muscles as you move down the back to the sacrum. Repeat, starting from the left-hand edge of the spine. Remember to get feedback from the recipient that your pressure is comfortable.

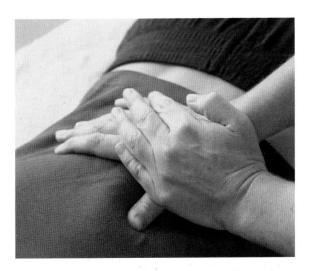

HAND ROLL DOWN THE BACK

6 **Stand on the left side of the recipient** and place the outside edge of your cupped right hand on your recipient's back. With a relaxed wrist flip your hand over – as it is flipping, your hand should open. This movement should be quick and smooth. Continue hand flips from the shoulders to the sacrum. Repeat several times.

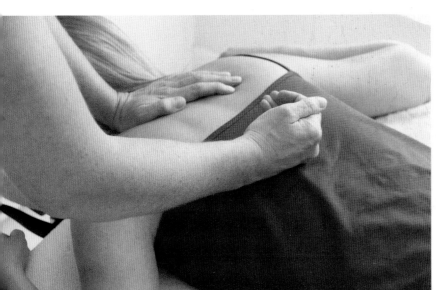

UPPER BODY STRETCH

7 Standing or kneeling on the right side of the recipient, place your right hand under the left shoulder and the heel of your left hand on the right side of the lower back.

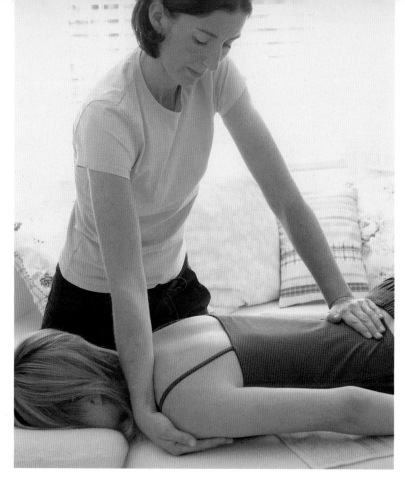

8 Lean back and slowly pull the shoulder up, while pushing the lower back away from the spine. Gently release. Never bounce or force a stretch.

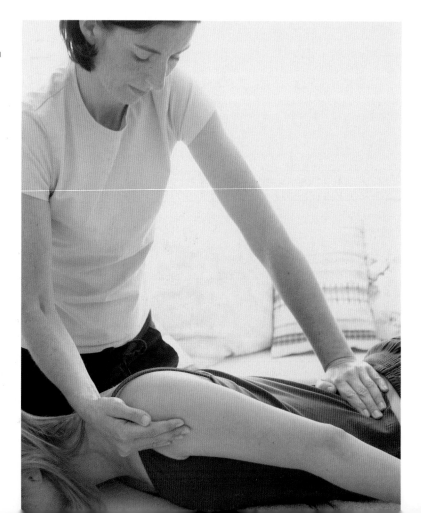

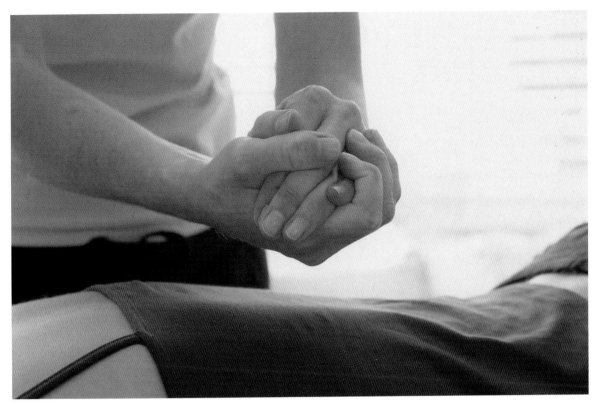

CUPPED-HAND PERCUSSION

9 **Cup your hands together, keeping the air inside.** With loose wrists, lightly strike the back. Work over both the shoulders and up and down the back. Do not apply cupped-hand percussion over the spine or any other bony area.

DOUBLE-HANDED PERCUSSION

10 **With loose wrists, relaxed fingers and your elbows out to the side,** apply light hacking movements to the body using alternate hands. Work over both the shoulders and up and down the back. Do not apply double-handed percussion over the spine or any other bony area.

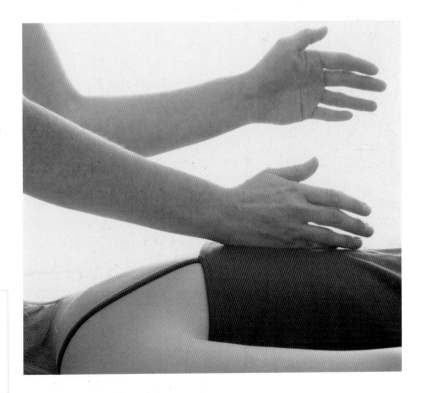

THE PERSON you have massaged will probably need at least a few minutes before they feel ready to get up. Help them to get up if necessary and advise them to drink plenty of water.

12.Ayurvedic massage

Ayurvedic massage is part of a detoxification and rejuvenation process used in Ayurvedic medicine – the other treatments of which are medicinal herbs, meditation, diet and yoga.

BACKGROUND

Ayurveda is an ancient Indian system of medicine dating back thousands of years. The term originates from the Sanskrit word "ayu", meaning life and "veda" meaning knowledge. Ayurvedic massage is concerned with maintaining and restoring mental and physical health. It is regarded as the forerunner of alternative medicine and promotes the belief that good health is the result of harmony between body, mind and spirit.

The system of Ayurveda is based on a thorough understanding of the energies of the five elements: ether, air, fire, water and earth, and the belief that every individual can be classified into three metabolic body types, known as "doshas". The three types are "vata", "pitta" and "kapha" and each one has distinctive characteristics. Everyone is born with a combination of the three doshas, but with one dominant. If this doshic constitution becomes imbalanced, illness may arise. Treatments include the use of medicinal herbs, meditation, diet, yoga and massage to bring about detoxification and rejuvenation. An Ayurvedic therapist will devise a customized program of treatment based on an individual's dosha type.

Here are some examples of Ayurvedic massage:
- ABHYANGA The most widely used full body massage where the type of oils, the speed and depth of treatment are dependent on the predominant dosha of the individual. Two practitioners may work in unison.
- URDVATHANA An invigorating massage using a herbal paste of grains, flour, herbs and oils to clean, tone and exfoliate the skin.
- SIRODHARA A method where a lukewarm trickle of oil is poured in a continuous stream on the forehead of the recipient for up to an hour.
- VISHESH An invigorating and deep massage.

TECHNIQUE

A professional Ayurvedic treatment can last from 45 to 90 minutes. The practitioner will take a thorough case history in order to work out a client's dosha type. Massage is given with the client undressed. The therapist will use warm sesame oil or an oil specifically chosen for that indivdual's dosha type. The massage techniques and depth will also vary according to the dosha type being treated.

Our guided massage provides a pampering and comforting self-help treatment. It is suitable for everyone, so your particular dosha doesn't need to be diagnosed by a professional practitioner. Following all the steps on a regular basis will help you to relax, aid detoxification and improve your skin quality.

You do not have to follow the sequence of the guided massage, you can do the treatment in the order you feel most comfortable. Try to make your techniques flow smoothly and direct your strokes in the direction of the heart when massaging your limbs.

Start by warming the sesame oil – in a bowl over a radiator or in a bowl sitting in hot water. Be careful not to heat the oil above a comfortable level. Sit or stand on a towel either naked or in your underwear. When you've completed the massage, leave the oil on your body for up to an hour before showering. Sesame oil will balance and calm the nervous system and is a nutrient for the skin.

Before you start the guided massage, consider whether any of the contraindications on page 10–11 apply to you. If you are confident there is no reason not to do these techniques, you can begin.

BENEFITS

Ayurvedic massage helps to relieve muscle tension and insomnia; it aids detoxification, and improves skin quality.

- ◆ **Vata: Slight frame, dry hair and skin, narrow nose and mouth, enthusiastic and energetic**
- ◆ **Pitta: Medium frame, fair with freckles or moles, fine hair, pointed nose and chin, impatient**
- ◆ **Kapha: Short with a large frame, pale, thick wavy hair, round face with large nose and mouth, relaxed and serene**

SCALP MASSAGE

1 **You may want to start your massage by sitting.** Apply some of the warmed oil to your hands and massage your scalp with your fingertips in firm circular movements as though washing the hair. Try to move the skin over the scalp and make your movements slow and rhythmical. Continue until you start to feel your scalp loosening under your fingers.

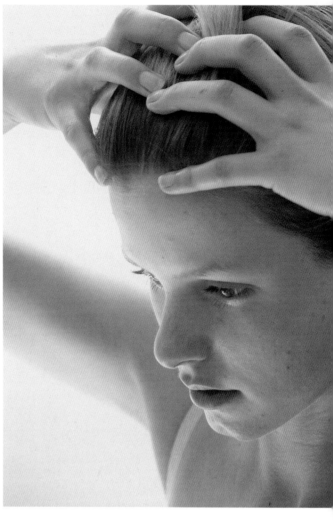

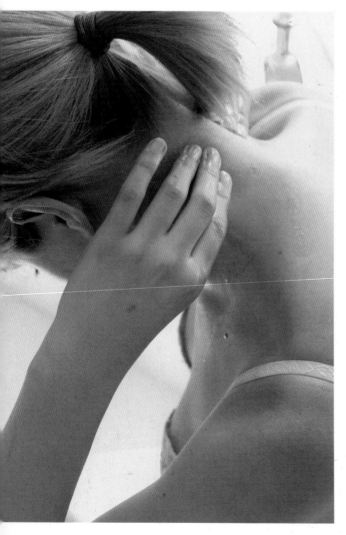

NECK MASSAGE

2 **Apply a little more oil to your hands if needed.** With your head bent slightly forwards, place your fingers behind your neck on the outside edge of the spine and squeeze the neck muscles between your fingers and palms. Work from the base of your neck to the base of your skull, circling around the base of the skull and then moving back down the neck. Repeat with your neck bent slightly back and in a neutral upright position.

SHOULDER MASSAGE

3 **Grip your shoulders between your thumbs and fingers or fingers and palms;** pull up and squeeze your muscles from the base of the neck to the shoulders. Repeat backwards and forwards along the shoulders until you start to feel the muscles relax. Grip the muscles at the top of your back with your fingertips and pull forwards and over the shoulders, before releasing. Repeat.

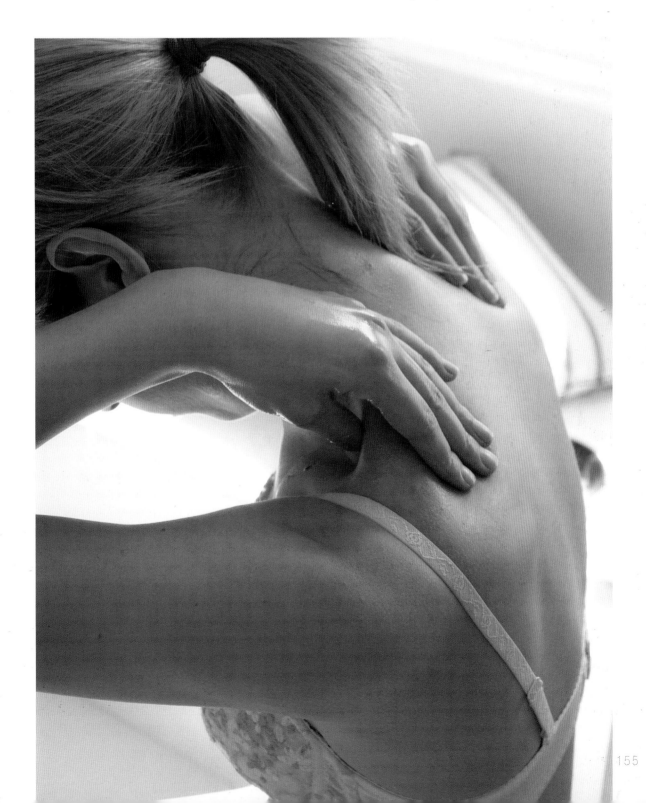

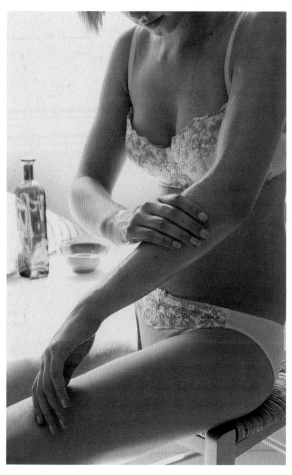

EFFLEURAGING FROM ARM TO SHOULDER

4 **Apply a little more oil to your hands** and make a sweeping effleurage stroke along one arm from wrist to shoulder and circle around the back of the shoulder. Repeat several times. Squeeze up the fleshy parts of your arm from the wrist to the shoulder and follow with effleurage.

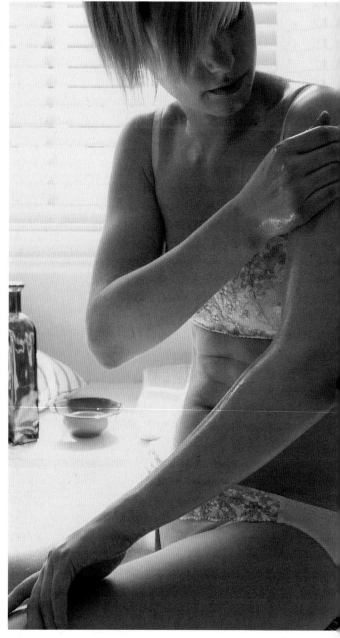

EFFLEURAGING FROM SHOULDER TO CHEST

5 **Apply more oil to your hand and pull your fingers down** from the top of the collarbone to the top of the breast. Push your fingers out towards the armpit, gently draw them back to the breast, push them back up the collarbone, circle around the shoulder and pull your hand back up over the shoulder. Repeat several times.

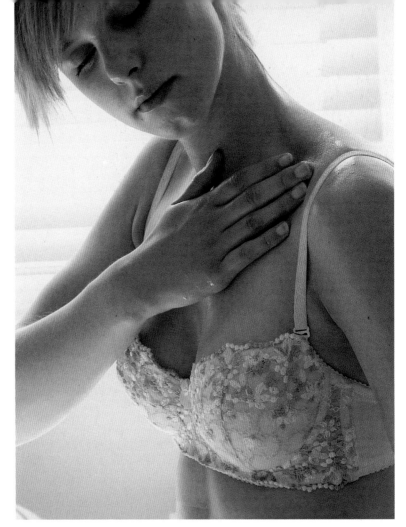

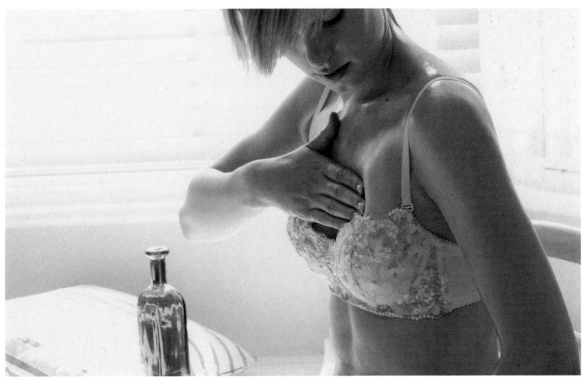

EFFLEURAGING
UP THE NECK

6 **Apply more oil to your hand
and effleurage** from the base
of the neck to one side of the chin.
Flick your fingers off the chin.
Repeat to cover front of the neck.
Repeat steps 4–6 on the other
arm, shoulder and neck.

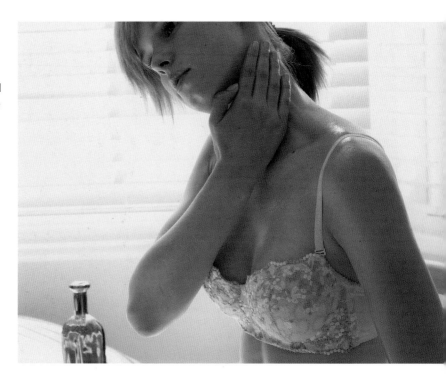

MASSAGING
THE NAVEL

7 **Stand up for the next steps.**
Apply oil to your hands and
gently sweep your right hand,
followed by your left hand, across
your stomach from left to right.
Pull your hands up the side of your
stomach and continue circling
around the navel in a clockwise
direction. Repeat up to five times.

EFFLEURAGING DOWN
THE BACK TO SACRUM

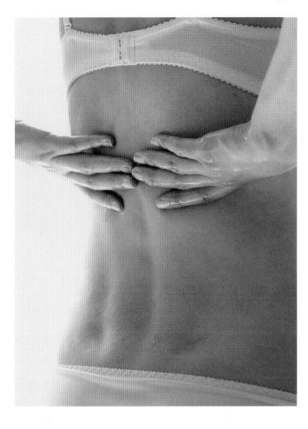

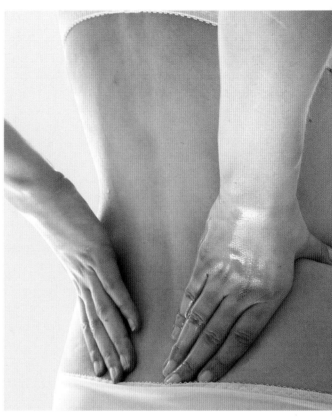

8 **Apply oil to your hands** and put them as far up your back as they will comfortably reach. Pull them down to your lower back.

PULLING ACROSS
THE LOWER BACK

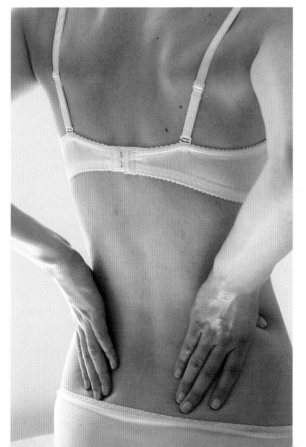

9 **From your lower back, pull your hands across to your sides.** Swing your hands up your back again and repeat steps 8 and 9 as many times as feels good.

MASSAGING OIL
INTO THE FEET

10 **You may want to sit with a stool in front of you for the final steps.** Apply more oil to your hands and massage oil into and around your feet.

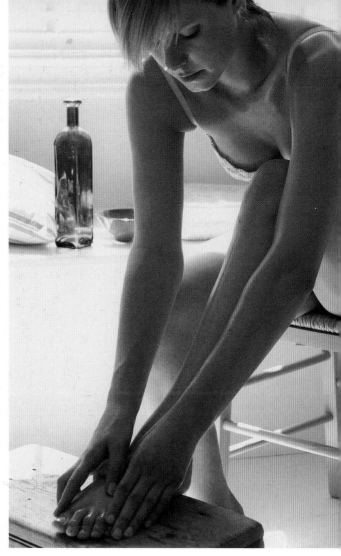

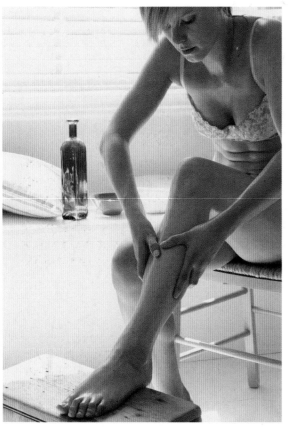

EFFLEURAGING FROM
FEET TO KNEES

11 **Apply more oil to your hands** and wrap them around your calf, pressing your fingers into the back of your calf muscle to pull up to your knee. Repeat.

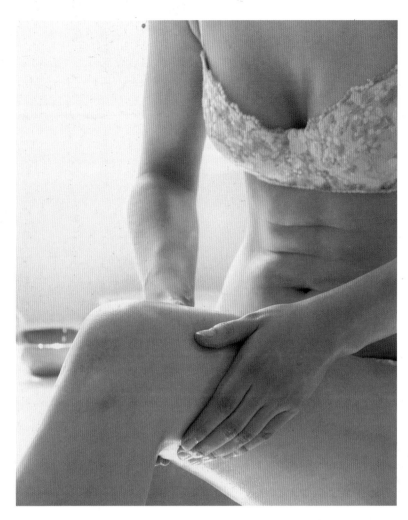

CRISS-CROSSING AND KNEADING THIGHS

12 **This step can be done either sitting or standing.** Apply more oil to your hands and wrap them around your thigh and pull up. Sweep your hands back to your knee and repeat. Now knead up the outside of your thigh.

Place your fingers behind your leg, just above the knee, pulling your fingers up through the muscles until your palms reach the top of the leg. Push your palms back down and repeat. Complete the leg massage with a couple of long effleurage strokes from the foot to the top of the thigh. Repeat steps 10–12 on the other leg.

MASSAGING YOUR HANDS

13 **Apply a little more oil to your hands** and rub them together as if applying hand cream. Use one thumb to massage in around the other thumb and across the palm of your other hand. Wiggle and pull each finger from the base to the tips, between your thumb and forefinger. Repeat on your other hand and thumb. Flick both of your hands to finish the treatment.

> **REMEMBER** to leave the sesame oil on your body for at least an hour before showering – it will help to calm the nervous system and is a nutrient for the skin.

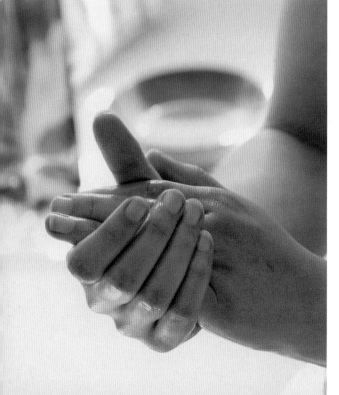

13. Thai massage

Thai massage includes palming, thumbing and assisted stretches, similar to those used in yoga.

BACKGROUND

Thai massage originated in India over 2,500 years ago as part of the ancient healing traditions of Ayurved. It is believed to have been developed by Jivaka Kumar Bhaccha, a friend and physician to the Buddha. Hence it is firmly embedded in the Buddhist philosophy and was practised and taught in Buddhist temples. It was embraced in Thailand following the spread of Buddhism throughout Southeast Asia.

The method is a synthesis of yoga, Ayurveda and meditation. It is also known as Thai yoga massage and "lazy man's yoga". There are two styles: the Northern school, more commonly practised in the West, is an energetic technique incorporating palming, thumbing and stretching; the Southern school works more specifically on different energy lines and is aimed at relaxation, but is not often practised in the West.

Thai massage views much illness as the result of imbalances between mind, body and spirit. It aims to rectify and balance any disharmony by working on the flow of life energy. In this therapy, the life energy is known as "prana" (the equivalent of ki in shiatsu). Like ki, prana circulates around the body through channels called "sen". There are 10 main channels, along which lie many acupoints, known as "marma". Thai massage works to relieve blockages or imbalances of prana by stimulating the sen and marma through pressure and assisted stretching in positions similar to yoga postures. It is thought this will improve health and wellbeing, and increase the overall flexibility of the skeletal structure.

TECHNIQUE

A professional Thai massage treatment will typically take 90 minutes. It will take place on a firm mat or futon on the floor. The recipient wears loose clothing, so oils are not used. The therapist will usually take a full case history prior to treatment. There is no set sequence and the client may be moved through several seated and lying positions. The techniques incorporate palming, thumbing and gentle passive and assisted stretches. An advanced

Thai practitioner may also use a technique called blood stopping. This involves the application of pressure at four major arteries to cleanse, revitalize and stimulate the flow of blood.

You can give your Thai massage on a futon or on a suitably padded floor. Both you and the person you are massaging should wear loose, comfortable clothing. Following the guided steps will take you approximately one hour. Try to follow the whole sequence to achieve maximum benefit. Make sure that you palm every muscle to warm it before going into the assisted stretches. Increase the pressure of your palming gradually as you work into areas of tension.

It is very important that all the stretches are increased progressively and are not held for too long; you must communicate with the person you are treating and never try to push the body beyond its limits.

The assisted stretching techniques are used to take the muscles through a full range of movements to increase their range of motion. Use your body weight to guide the recipient into the postures. It is very important that the stretches are increased progressively and are not held for too long; you must communicate with the person you are massaging and never try to push the body beyond its boundaries. Make sure all your techniques flow smoothly and are applied with sensitivity. Encourage the person you are treating to relax, breathe deeply and to exhale as you apply pressure or take a muscle into a stretch.

Before you start the guided massage, you should have run through the list of contraindications on page 10–11 with the person you are going to treat. Note that only a professional therapist should treat a pregnant woman. If you are both confident that there is no reason why the treatment should not be given, you can begin.

BENEFITS

Thai massage helps to stretch and tone the muscles, improves the circulation, relieves tension, boosts the immune system and balances the body's energy.

SHOULDER
PALMING

1 **The recipient should sit cross-legged,** hands in lap. Stand behind and place your hands on the shoulders. Place your palms at the neck/shoulder junction and your fingers over the shoulders. Alternately apply pressure through your palms to massage their shoulders from the neck out. Repeat.

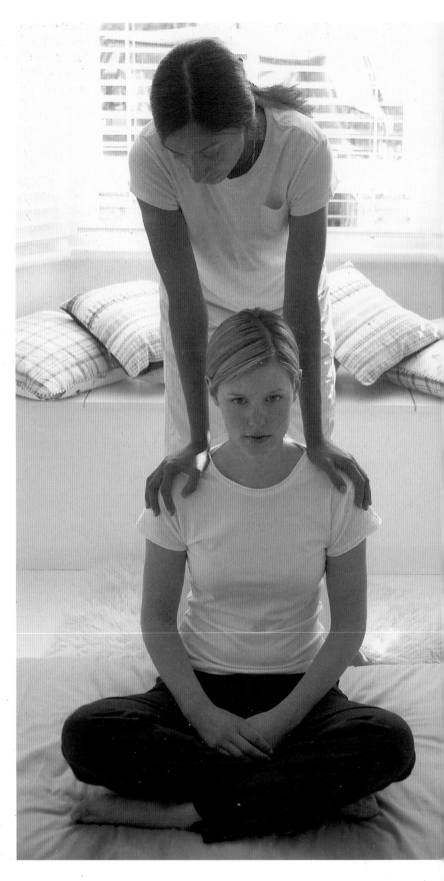

SHOULDER ROLLING

2 Kneel behind the recipient and rest your left hand on the left shoulder.

Place the fleshiest part of your right forearm (palm down) on to the right shoulder and, starting at the neck/shoulder junction, press your forearm down and roll it out so that the palm turns upwards. Continue to the end of the shoulder. Repeat on the left shoulder, resting on the right.

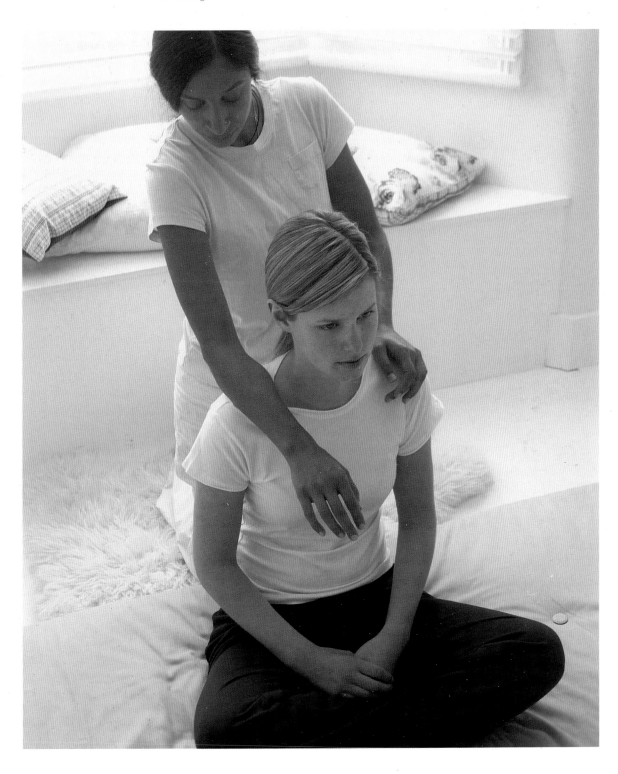

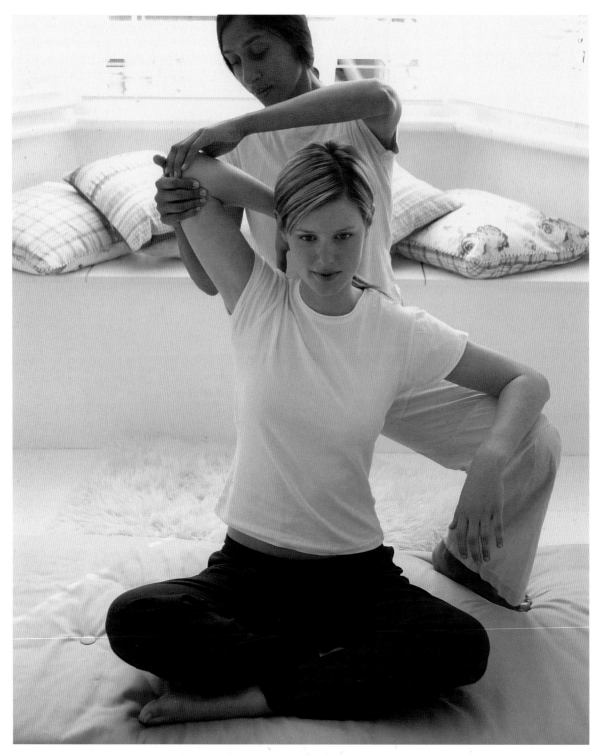

ARM STRETCH

3 **Kneel behind your recipient and raise one leg.** Rest one of the recipient's arms on your raised leg to provide postural support. Grasp the other arm by the elbow and wrist and slowly lift it above behind the head so that the forearm dangles down the back. Squeeze the muscles between the elbow and armpit. Release and guide the arm slowly back. Never over-extend the arm or squeeze the muscles too vigorously.

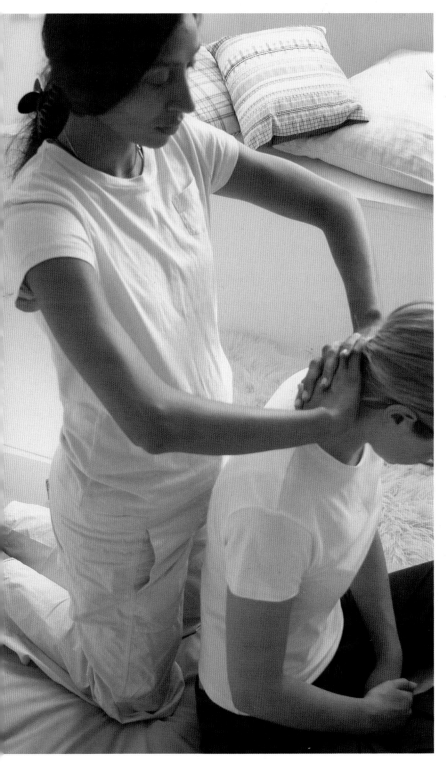

NECK PALMING

4 **Kneel behind the recipient,** whose head should be dropped slightly down. Interlace your fingers and place your palms either side of the neck to squeeze the neck muscles with the heels of the hands. Work up and down the neck. Repeat several times.

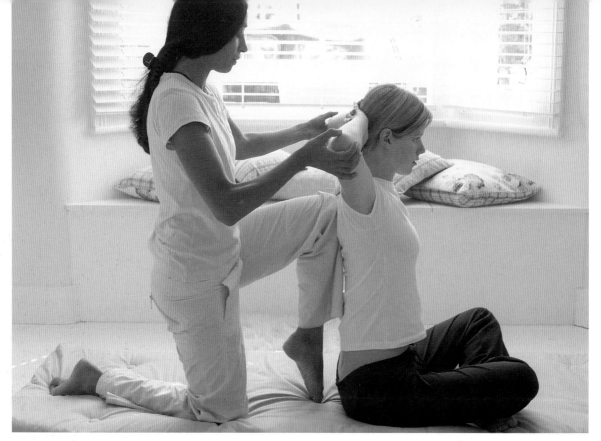

SHOULDER AND ARM STRETCH

5 **Kneel behind the recipient with one leg raised to support the back.** Grasp the arms by the elbows and lift them outwards and upwards. Ask the recipient to lock hands behind the head. Slide your hands to the front of their elbows and hold.

Gently stretch the elbows out to the side and back and hold for up to 30 seconds. Release and guide the arms back to the sides of the body.

PALMING THE INSTEPS OF THE FOOT

6 **Ask the recipient to lie down on their back** with legs shoulder width apart and feet pointing out. Palm all over one foot with the heel of your hand. Repeat on the other foot.

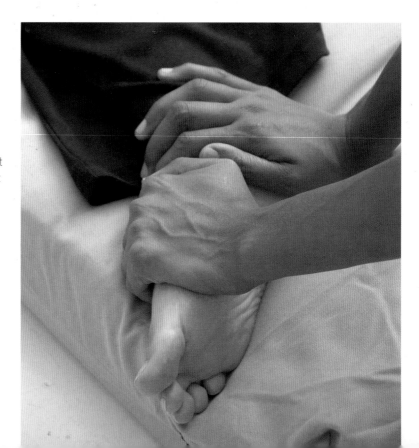

THE TREE STRETCH

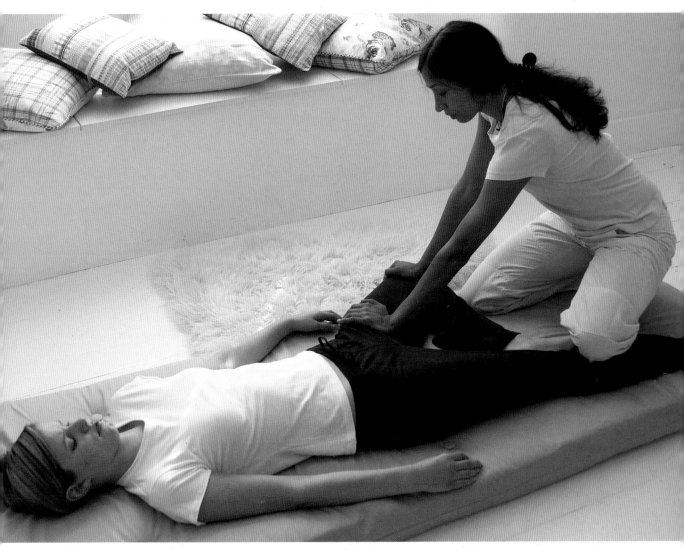

7 **Palm up the inside of one leg from the ankle to the knee.**
Palm up the inside, middle and outside of the leg from the knee to
the thigh. Take the recipient's foot and bend it towards the inner thigh.
Secure the knee at the floor with one hand and palm up and down the
inner thigh with the other. Repeat on the other leg.

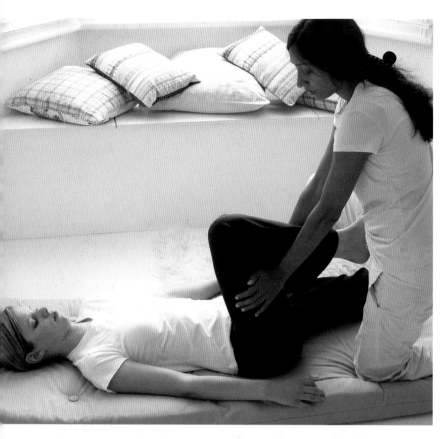

HAMSTRING STRETCH

8 **You should be positioned with one of your knees on the floor** (about level with your recipient's knee) and the other leg raised and stretched across the recipient's body. Ask the recipient to bend one knee and raise it, so that the foot is resting just above your groin area. Support the leg by placing your hands around the back of the thigh. This is where three large muscles, jointly known as the hamstrings, are situated.

PALMING THE STRETCHED HAMSTRING

9 **Use your body weight to slowly push the leg towards the chest.** Hold the position in mid-stretch and palm up and down their hamstrings. Gently release the leg and slowly lower it back on to the futon or floor. Do not overstretch or overwork the hamstrings. Always check that your recipient feels comfortable before continuing. Repeat on the other leg.

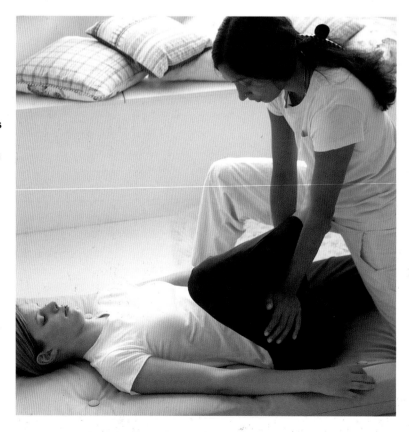

ARMS, LEGS AND TORSO STRETCH

10 **Kneel behind the recipient's head,** take hold of the wrists and gradually move the arms above their head. Raise the arms very slightly and lean back to stretch the arms, torso and legs. Hold the stretch for 30 seconds, before releasing and lowering the arms. Rest for 10 seconds. Repeat three times.

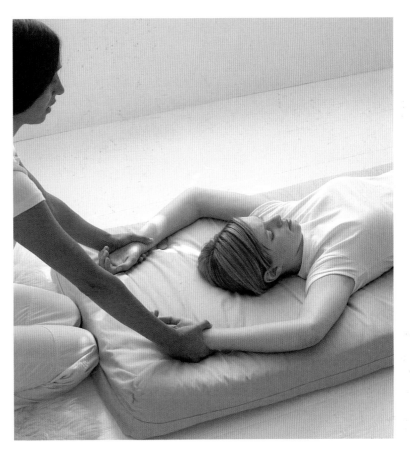

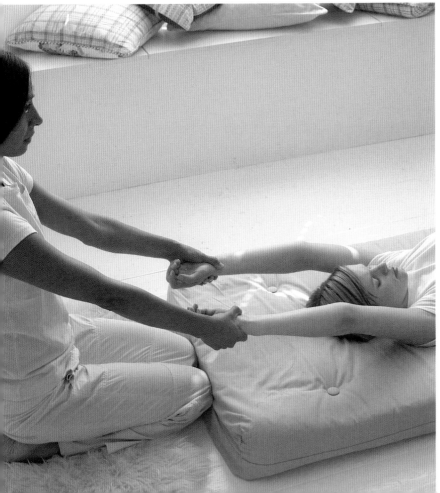

THE PERSON you have massaged will probably need at least a few minutes before they feel ready to get up. Help them to get up if necessary and advise them to drink plenty of water.

14. Lymphatic drainage

A treatment that will stimulate your lymphatic system and boost a sluggish circulation.

BACKGROUND

Lymphatic drainage is a form of massage that aims to stimulate and improve the circulation of the lymphatic system in the body. The lymphatic system drains excess fluid from the spaces around the tissues and transports this fluid (known as lymph) to the lymph nodes, which filter it to remove waste, harmful cells, bacteria and toxins. The remaining lymph re-enters the cardiovascular system and the cycle is repeated.

The lymphatic system also protects against infection by producing antibodies and white blood cells. The main lymph nodes are found in the neck, armpits, groin, behind the knees and on the inside of the elbows. Lymph is collected into two main channels before rejoining the body's circulation: the thoracic duct receives lymph from the left side of the head, neck and chest, the left arm and the lower limbs. The right lymphatic duct drains lymph from the right side of the head, neck, chest and the right arm.

The lymphatic system depends on muscular contraction, gravity and passive movement to push lymph through the lymph vessels to the lymph nodes. Inactivity and muscle tension will hinder its flow. The techniques applied in lymphatic drainage massage are designed to stimulate the movement of lymphatic fluids in order to assist the body in cleansing and elimination of waste products. Manual lymphatic drainage is an advanced form of lymphatic drainage and was founded by Dr Emil Vodder, a Danish biologist, in the 1930s. It is similar to lymphatic drainage, but the therapists are highly trained to treat conditions from general sluggish circulation to lymphoedema in cancer patients.

TECHNIQUE

A professional treatment will take between 30 and 90 minutes. A thorough case history is taken prior to the treatment. The massage will take place on a massage table with the recipient undressed. No oil is used. The massage techniques are slow, light and very specific. They incorporate rhythmical pumping, effleurage and stationary circular movements with the pads of the fingers, thumb and the palms of the hands to manually push fluid towards the nodes. A treatment will generally begin with the lymph nodes in the neck, followed by the chest, arms, legs, back and stomach; and returning to the neck to finish.

Our guided massage provides a self-help treatment to aid your lymphatic system and boost a sluggish circulation. It is important that you follow the order and sequence of the massage to gain maximum benefit. You should always drain the area nearest the topmost node first to clear a path for the lymphatic fluid to move up from other areas. Lymph must be pushed up the body towards a node. Lymph flowing backwards will cause no harm but will not benefit you.

Use very slow and gentle pressure in soft pumping, scooping and circular movements. If your skin reddens you are applying too much pressure, which can cause blockages, pain and fluid build-up. Your skin will move, but be careful not to drag it.

Before you start the guided massage, consider whether any of the contraindications on page 10–11 apply to you. You must be sure that any minor puffiness or swelling is not the result of a medical condition. Do not treat yourself if you suffer from diabetes, kidney, liver or heart disease or cancer. If you are in any doubt, consult your doctor. If you are confident that there is no reason not to do these techniques, you can begin.

Dry body brushing enhances lymphatic drainage, aiding detoxification and promoting natural healing. Try to body brush every day for five weeks and thereafter three times a week.

BENEFITS

Lymphatic massage boosts the immune and lymphatic systems and enhances energy. By releasing congestion, swelling and fluid retention, it can improve the appearance of the skin and aid recuperation from illness.

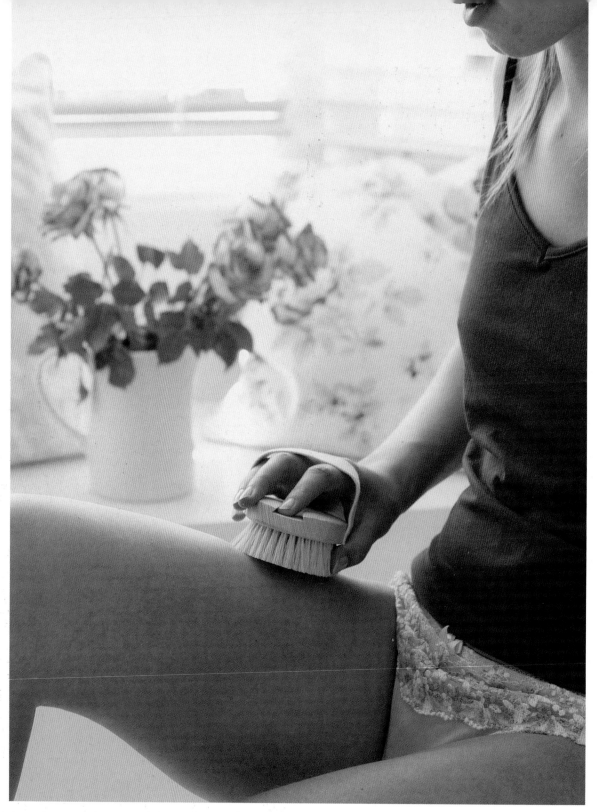

BODY BRUSHING

1 **You will need to buy a soft bristle brush** (available from most chemists and health stores). Either sitting or standing, dry brush your legs with the brush – starting at the ankles and gradually moving up to the top of your thigh. Brush from the inside of your leg to the middle, outside and around the back. Brush lightly to avoid scratching your skin. Repeat on other leg.

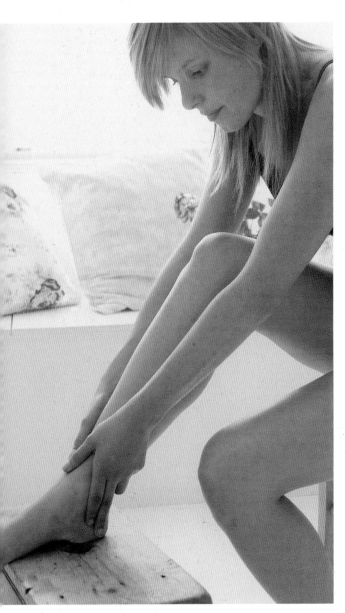

EFFLEURAGE

2 **Wrap your hands around your calf** and, using long sweeping strokes, effleurage up from your ankle to the top of your thigh. Repeat until every area of your leg has been effleuraged.

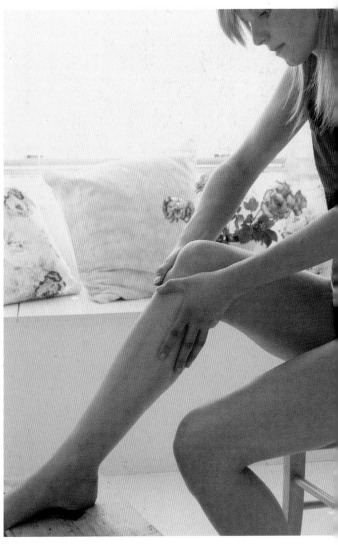

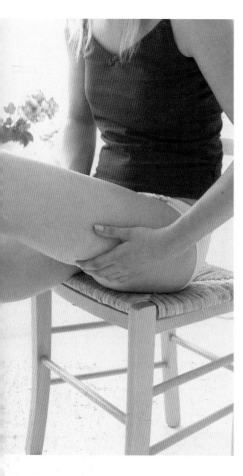

PUMPING

3 **With one knee bent and slightly raised,** place your hands under the top of your thigh. Apply small circles, moving the skin towards the lymph nodes in the groin – your skin should move without you fingers sliding across it. Continue circling down your leg to the back of the knee. Follow with effleurage from the back of the leg up to the groin.

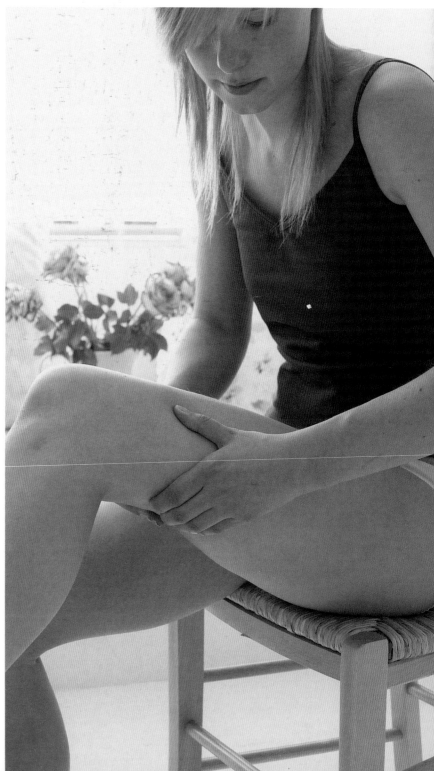

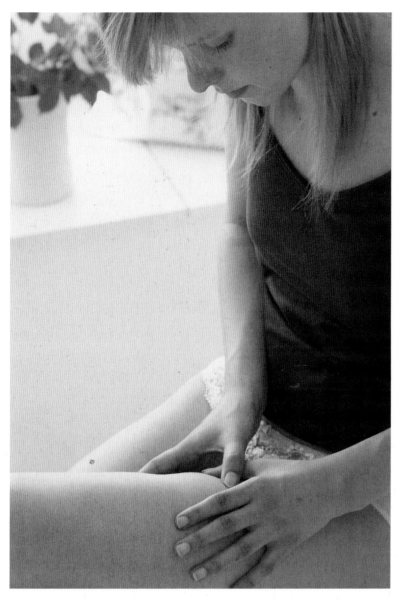

PUMPING CIRCLES

4 **Place your hands on top of one thigh** – your fingers pointing towards your knee. Massage in a semi-circle sweeping your fingers around – as if you were pushing the lymph up the leg. Start at the top of your thigh and work down to the knee. Follow with effleurage.

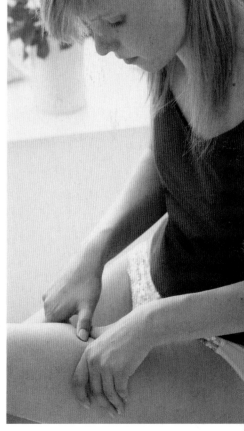

CIRCLING
THE KNEE

5 **Place your fingers on your knee and massage** around your kneecap in small finger circles. Move your fingers gently towards the back of the knee – to flush the lymph to the knee node.

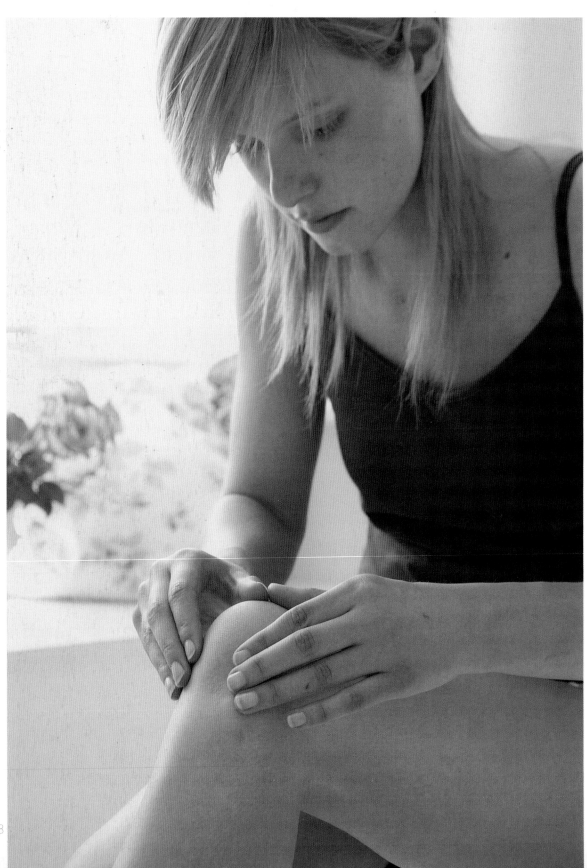

CLEARING THE KNEE NODE

6 **Apply gentle semi-circular** strokes behind your knee and then effleurage up to the groin.

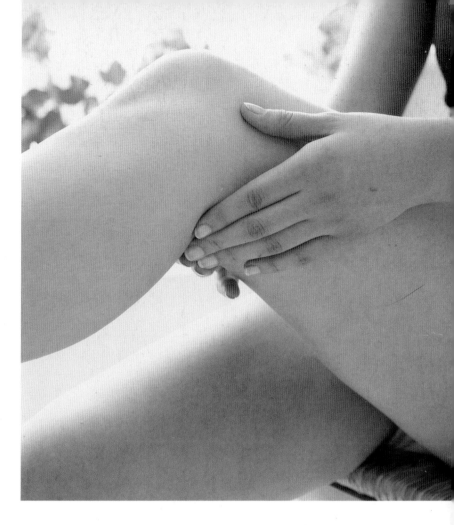

CALF EFFLEURAGE

7 **Wrap your hands around your ankle** and effleurage up the calf to the knee node.

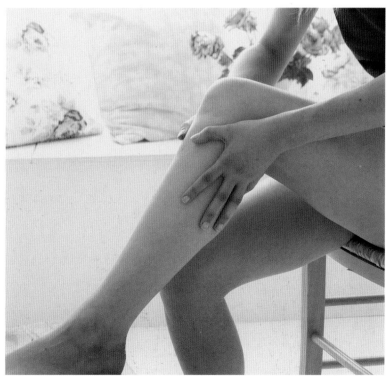

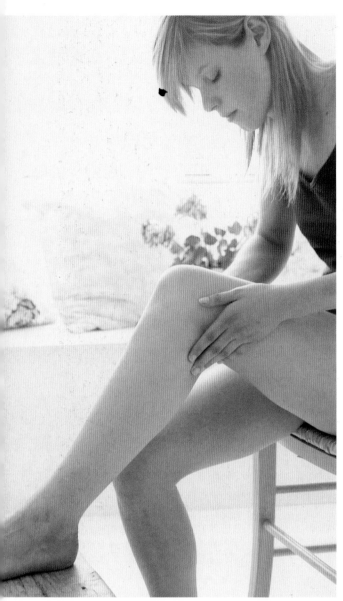

CALF CIRCLES

8 **Starting just below your knee,** use semi-circular pumping strokes around the calf and up to the knee node. Repeat this technique down your leg until you reach the ankle. Wrap your hands around your calf and gently effleurage up to the knee.

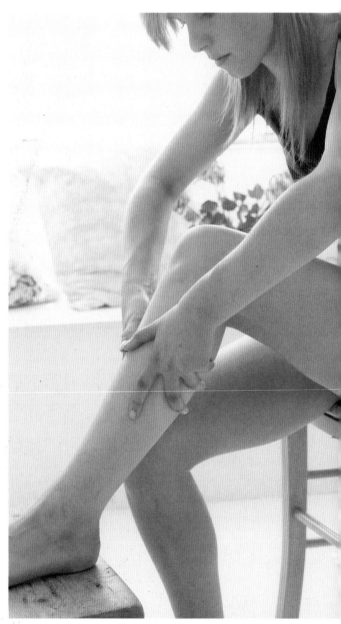

ANKLE CIRCLES

9 **Starting at the top of your foot,** effleurage around your ankle with your fingers. Repeat a couple of times. Now apply small, circular pumping strokes around the ankle and flush up the Achilles tendon to the knee node. Repeat three times.

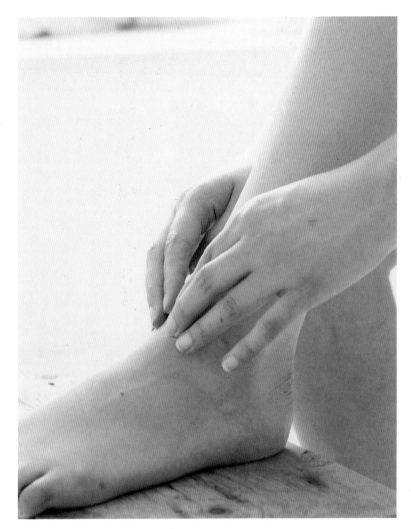

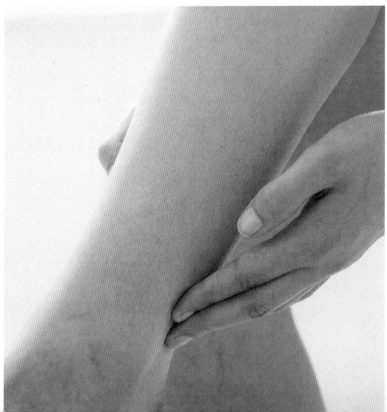

FINAL EFFLEURAGE FLUSH

10 Finish the treatment with three long effleurage strokes from your foot, right up to your groin. Continue until your have covered every area of your leg. Repeat all the steps on the other leg.

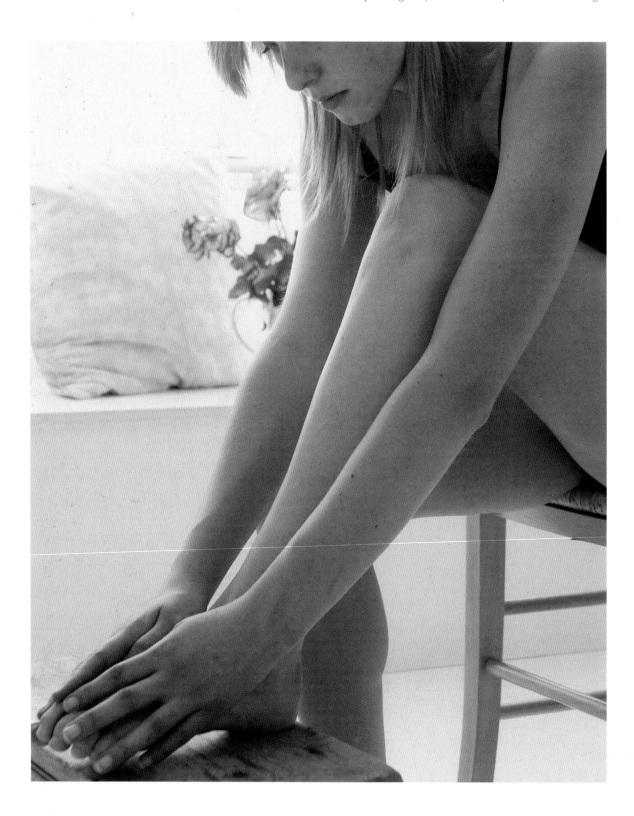

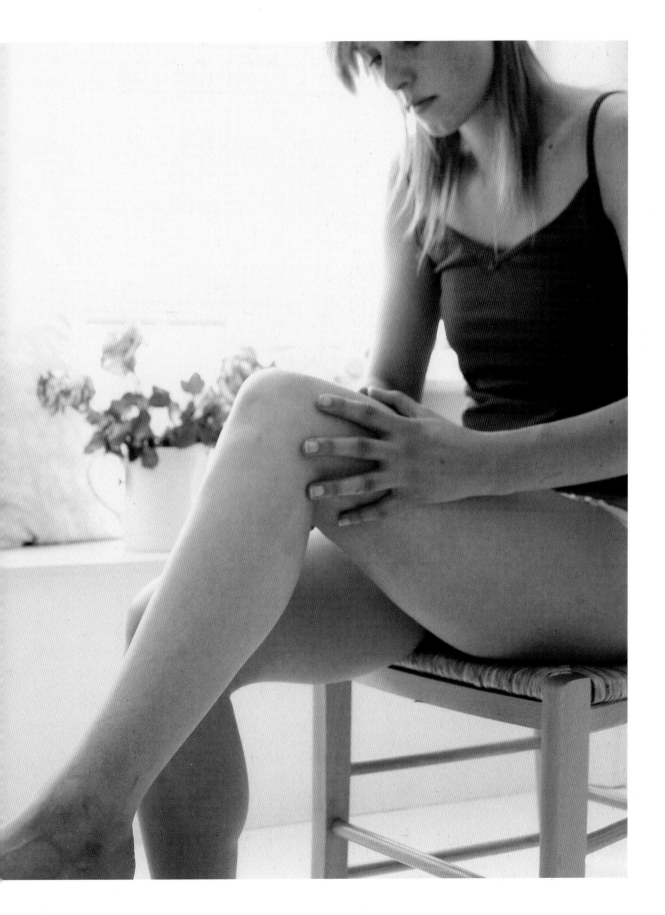

15.Partner massage

Partner massage is a wonderful way to show love and helps couples to increase their intimacy and communication.

BACKGROUND

Massage is not only an aid to relieve stress, aches and pains, but it is also a wonderful means of communication between two people. Giving and receiving a massage can help to maintain a loving, caring relationship between a couple, and may even help to revive a troubled relationship. In the Hindu tradition, massage is an important ritual before a marriage takes place. In India and Africa and many other cultures, massage is used as a means to help conception.

In a world where most people live busy and stressful lives, it is good to stop, close the door and get away from all distractions, such as the TV and computers – simply to give or receive a massage with your partner. This quiet time together as a couple is precious: it allows for intimacy, communication, love and sympathy – all of the things that we sometimes forget to give the person we love. Massage is a great way to develop awareness of each other's mental and physical state, as well as supporting a partner who may be feeling anxious, tired or run down.

TREATMENT

The steps in our guided partner massage are based on Swedish techniques, with the addition of lots of light feathery effleurage strokes to areas of heightened sensitivity – the inner thigh, stomach, lower back, inner arms, ears, neck, face, lips and feet.

Following all the steps in the massage sequence will take approximately an hour. You may choose to do a shorter massage; it is up to you and will be dependent on the time you have and your energy levels. You may also decide to use some of the other techniques that have been covered in this book. Find out how your partner is feeling and what sort of treatment they would like.

Whether you are giving a deep, penetrating massage or a reflexology treatment, try to make your sequence flow smoothly. Run your hands around the contours of your partner's body and seduce him or her with your touch. Experiment, map out your partner's sensual areas and, most of all, use your imagination and have fun.

Before you start your massage, why not set the scene to help make the experience even more intimate? Dim the lights, light a candle and play some relaxing music. You could use an aphrodisiac blend of essential oils such as rose, neroli, ylang ylang or patchouli in a carrier massage oil or in a burner.

Before you start the guided massage, you should have run through the list of contraindications on page 10–11 with the person you are going to treat. If you are both confident that there is no reason why the treatment should not be given, you can begin.

BENEFITS

Massage between couples can be purely for fun and relaxation, but it can also be highly sensual and erotic and may therefore aid those couples who are experiencing difficulties with sexual intimacy. Massaging each other for just 10 minutes every day can be enormously beneficial.

Massaging your partner is a great way to develop awareness of each other's mental and physical state, as well as supporting a partner who may be feeling anxious or run down.

FEATHER STROKES

1 **Start with your partner lying face down** and sit astride your partner's hips or, alternatively, you may prefer to sit by their side. Follow steps 1–8 from the Swedish massage (see pages 38–42). Place your fingers on either side of the spine and, with light, feathery strokes, move them down the back from the neck to the sacrum. Allow one hand to follow the other as you repeat. Try not to tickle your partner and pay special attention to any areas of heightened sensitivity, for example, the sacrum and the neck.

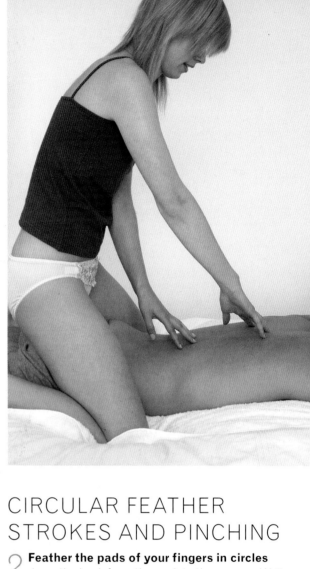

CIRCULAR FEATHER STROKES AND PINCHING

2 **Feather the pads of your fingers in circles** down the back from the neck to the sacrum. Write little notes on your partners back with the pads of your fingers. Gently pinch small areas of skin between your thumb and forefinger to heighten the sensitivity of the skin. Have fun and elaborate.

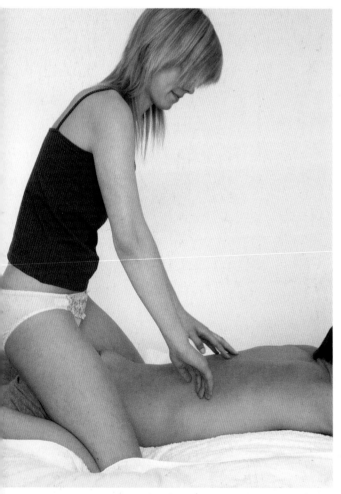

SACRUM MASSAGE

3 **Gently massage around the sacrum and the top of the buttocks** with the pads of your fingers or thumbs. Dance the pads of your fingers around in gentle feathery strokes and tease the skin of this highly sensitive area with your touch.

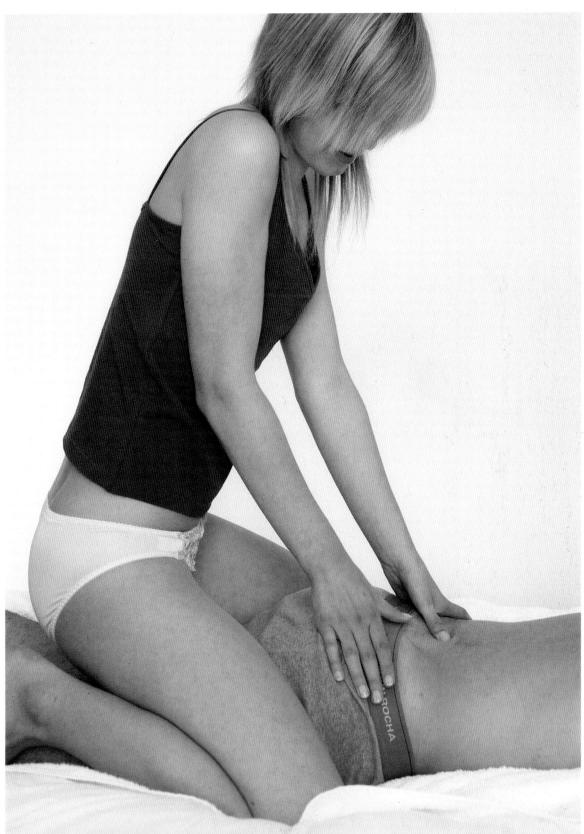

LEG MASSAGE

4 **Massage the leg using steps 11–12 of Swedish massage** (see page 44). Pay special attention to the inner thigh. Pull your hands up through the inner thigh and around the buttocks. Repeat, fanning and dancing your hand in and out of the thigh in circles.

Stroke down the leg massage to the calf and slowly pull your hands off at the foot.

Repeat on the other leg. Now ask your partner to turn onto their front.

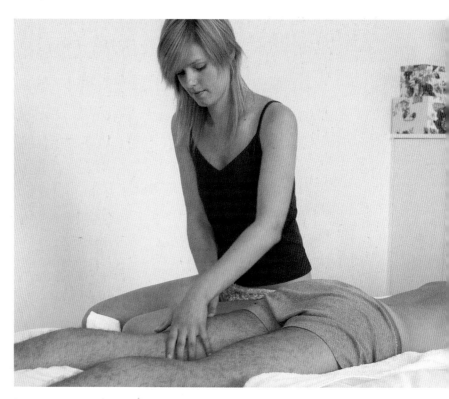

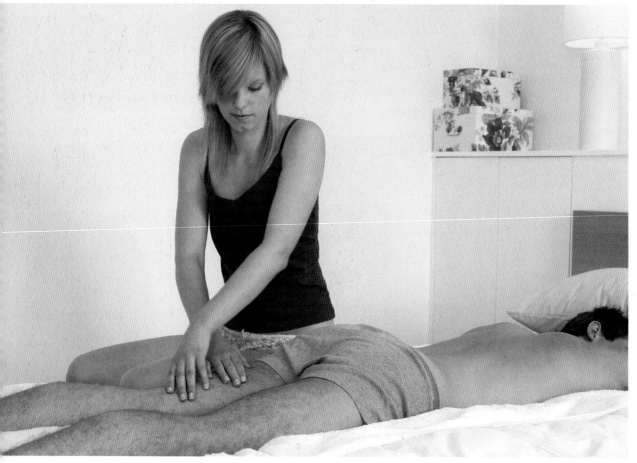

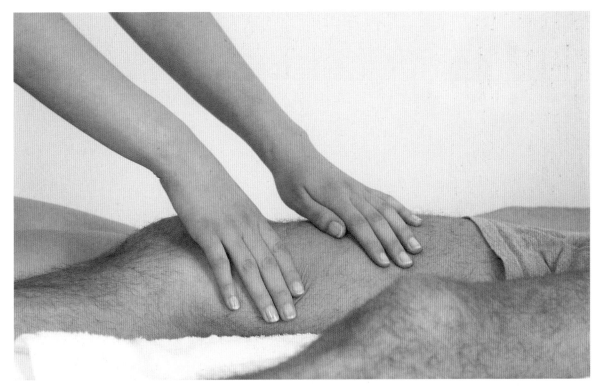

LEG MASSAGE

5 **Spread your partner's leg out** and feather the pads of your fingertips up through their inner thigh. Stroke up the inner thigh, lightly moving your fingers around the groin region and feather back down to the knee. Have fun and continue repeating the movements, asking your partner if there are any that he or she is particularly enjoying. Stroke down the calf and spend time massaging your partner's foot (see steps 18–19 from Swedish massage, pages 47–48). Repeat on the other leg.

ABDOMEN MASSAGE

6 **Place your fingers next to your partner's left hipbone** and feather across the abdomen to the right hipbone. Repeat with circular and wavy massage movements.

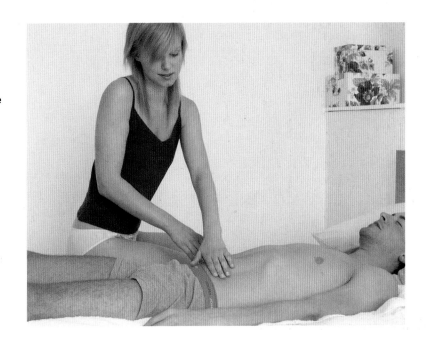

ABDOMEN MASSAGE

7 **From the right hipbone draw your fingers up and around the abdomen** in a clockwise direction. Try to use your hands alternately, with one following the other. You will be able to make a full circle with one hand and half a circle with the other, lifting one as it crosses the other. Continue with one hand making small circles.

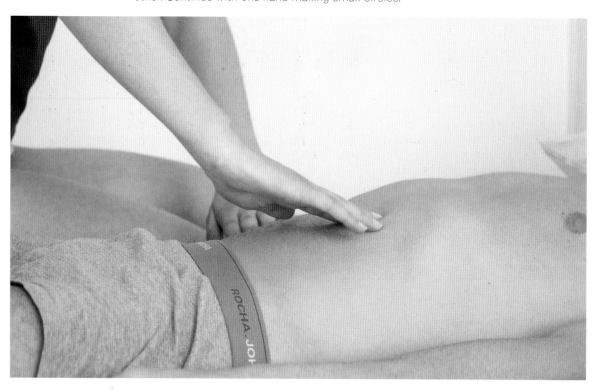

CHEST MASSAGE

8 **Draw your fingers down the front of your partner's chest** from the breastbone (sternum), fanning them out across the bottom of the ribs and down the sides of the body, before pulling your hands up either side of the abdomen. Repeat several times.

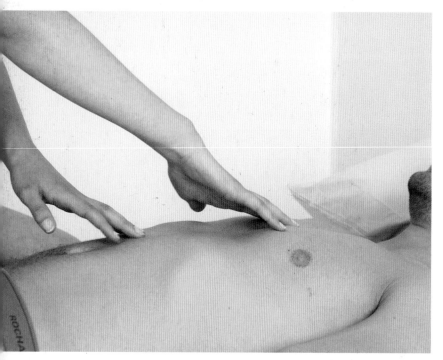

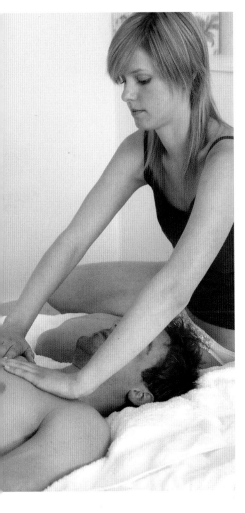

CHEST MASSAGE

9 **Sit at the top of your partner's head** and place your hands on the top of the chest. Stroke outwards to the shoulders and gently push them down to apply a stretch. Repeat. Return your hands to the top of the chest to effleurage down the sternum, before pulling your fingers back up around the chest. Lightly circle the chest and breast area until you reach the nipples. Experiment with increasing and decreasing the depth of your touch.

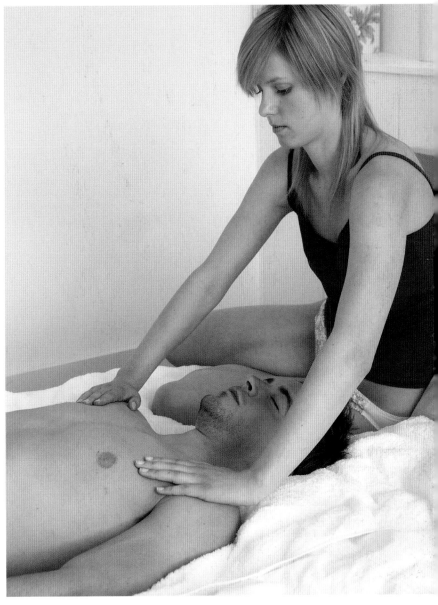

SQUEEZING AND FEATHERING THE ARM

10 **Squeeze the fleshy areas** of the tops of your partner's arms. Push your hands down the sides of the arms to the wrists and repeat. Do feather strokes up from the forearm to the armpit. Repeat with wave and circle movements.

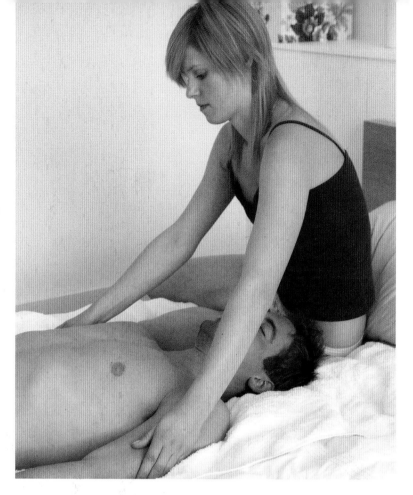

SHOULDER MASSAGE

11 **With your hands on the elbows,** pull up the outside of the arms, moving your hands under the shoulders and up towards the base of the neck. When you reach the base of the skull, push your hands back down the neck and across the shoulders to reach the elbows again. Repeat five times. This movement should feel like a great stretch and will bring most people up in goose bumps.

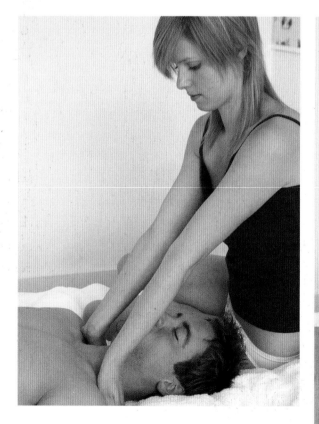

SCALP MASSAGE

12 **Start with the highly sensuous ears.** Squeeze each earlobe several times and then massage gently in and around the ear. Pull your hands up through the hairline onto the top of the scalp and massage the scalp with your fingers as if you were washing the hair. Repeat for several minutes (or longer if your partner wishes) and then gently pull little shafts of hair away from the scalp.

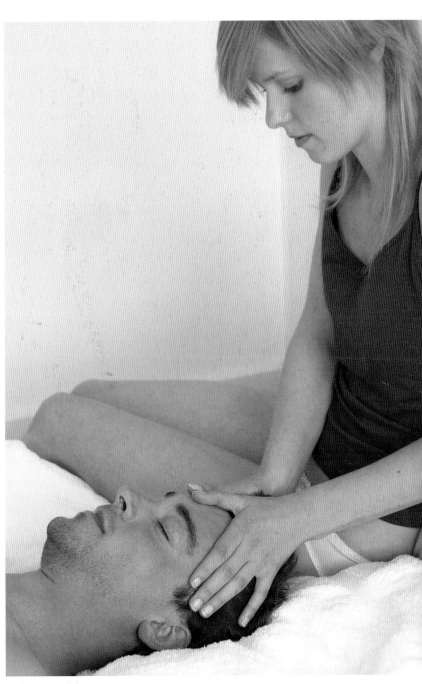

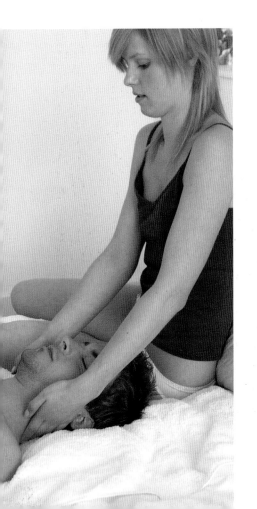

FINISH THE TREATMENT by feathering the pads of your fingers up and around your partner's face, paying special attention to the sensitive lips.

3

OTHER STYLES OF BODYWORK

Lomi lomi
(Hawaiian massage)

BACKGROUND

Lomi lomi is Hawaiian for "rub rub". It is an ancient practice of massage handed down through generations by native Hawaiian Shaman or Kahuna. Lomi lomi is a form of massage used to activate an inner state of self-realization, similar to that attained in deep meditation. Lomi lomi combines prayer and tne acknowledgment of the existence of a higher power along with "ku" or intuition, as an integral part of its technique.

It is based on a therapist using their subconscious mind to read the recipient's body's subtle vibrations and frequencies. The massage is spontaneous and its purpose is to bring alignment back to an individual's body, mind and spirit. A lomi lomi treatment begins and ends with a chant. Before it begins, the recipient is asked if they have any issues they want to resolve. They are asked to identify their issue with a symbol and to choose another positive symbol to represent how they would like it to be resolved. During the massage the recipient will alternate these symbols in their mind with the massage ending on the positive symbol.

TECHNIQUE

A Lomi lomi treatment lasts between two and three hours. It is carried out on a massage couch or floor mat. Oil is used to apply long, flowing choreographed strokes with the hands and forearms. Gentle neck and joint stretches are used to open and eliminate energy blockages. Lomi lomi techniques are energetic, vibrant and deeply relaxing.

BENEFITS

Lomi lomi soothes tired muscles and releases blocked emotions and unwanted thought patterns.

Polarity therapy

BACKGROUND

Polarity therapy was developed in the United States by Dr Randolph Stone in the 1940s. It is a method of bodywork that blends both Eastern and Western concepts of health to help the body heal itself. It is based on the theory that the life energy in our bodies is governed by positive and negative poles. These poles are complementary and necessary to each other, with equilibrium of mind, body and spirit being dependent on their harmonious interaction. It is believed that disease arises out of an imbalance between them. Polarity therapy aims to balance the flow of energy by massage, diet, exercise and counselling, thereby releasing any blockages and completing the energy circuit.

TECHNIQUE

A professional treatment will last approximately one hour. The first treatment will be based on taking a thorough case history of the physical, mental and dietary habits of the recipient through discussion, visual inspection and a gentle hands-on assessment of the energy flow and circulation in their body. Follow-up treatments will take place on a massage table and will be performed through the clothes. The therapist will work with the needs of the individual and will incorporate acupressure-style massage, chakra balancing and manipulation. Dietary changes and yoga exercises will be recommended to detoxify the system.

BENEFITS

Polarity therapy is intended to prevent illness by improving the circulation and immune system and aid stress-related conditions.

Bowen technique

BACKGROUND

The Bowen technique is a soft tissue remedial therapy that was developed in the 1950s by the Australian Thomas Bowen. It is a gentle and precise form of bodywork that uses the fingers and thumbs to apply rolling techniques, which are carried out in a specific sequence at key structural points – over soft tissue, tendons and ligaments – to stimulate the body's own healing mechanisms.

Bowen therapists follow the maxim that "less is more". The treatment is given in sets with regular two-minute breaks to allow the brain to register the status of the muscle, tendon or ligament and send information back down the spinal cord to the area being treated, at which point the body will respond and relax.

The breaks are vital to the success of the treatment. If there is no break, the brain will not be able to process all the related sensory information and the desired effect cannot be achieved. Two to three treatments may be recommended within a short time. Clients are also advised not to have any other forms of bodywork, massage, osteopathy or chiropracty whilst undergoing Bowen treatments.

TECHNIQUE

The treatment takes place with the recipient seated or lying on a massage table or bed. It is applied through loose clothing and will not involve the use of oils. A treatment will start with two stopper moves. Stoppers are used to open, assess and relax the body. These stoppers are located on the lower and upper back. A two minute break will then be taken before the treatment.

BENEFITS

The Bowen technique addresses many conditions, including anxiety, back pain, digestive disorders, migraines, respiratory problems and joint problems.

Feldenkrais

BACKGROUND

This method was developed by the atomic physicist and judo black belt – Moshe Feldenkrais. He combined his scientific knowledge with the Eastern philosophies of judo to create a method of movement designed to increase self-awareness and improve postural alignment and general health. Feldenkrais believed that posture and movement were one of the best indicators of an individual's thoughts and emotions.

He based his teachings on the importance of people being aware of and listening to their bodies. When muscles are balanced and relaxed, the body works in unison. If one muscle is not working correctly and another is over-compensating, it can result in postural imbalances, tension and possible injury. Feldenkrais believed that movements should be graceful and that this in turn would improve the structural and emotional wellbeing of an individual.

TECHNIQUE

There are two components to Feldenkrais:

◆ Awareness through movement – group classes in which a sequence of gentle movements are taught to raise awareness and function. Group classes lasting approximately one hour will generally involve lying and/ or sitting.

◆ Functional integration – one-on-one sessions tailored to the needs of the individual. The therapist will use his or her hands to take the recipient through guided movements; there is no tissue manipulation. These sessions usually take place on a massage table or chair, or standing.

BENEFITS

Feldenkrais aims to raise anatomical awareness, skeletal realignment, reduce pain and increase strength and co-ordination.

Rolfing

BACKGROUND

Rolfing was created in the United States by Doctor Ida Rolf. It is a deep tissue massage that is used to restore vertical alignment and rebalance the body.

Ida Rolf believed that physical and emotional stresses that cause a restriction or dysfunction in one area of the body will result in an overload or dysfunction in an adjacent area. Any imbalance will have a negative effect on the postural muscles and may affect the health and wellbeing of an individual. Rolfing aims to bring the posture back into its natural alignment. The result will be fluid movement, better posture and increased vitality.

TECHNIQUE

Rolfing treatment is usually given in 10 one-hour sessions. The treatment will take place on a massage couch. The massage will involve deep tissue manipulation applied through the fingers, knuckles and elbows, in order to stretch and relax the muscles, the connective tissue that encases muscle (fascia), bone, organs, nerves and blood vessels.

Rolfing may release past issues and traumas that have become embedded in the structure of the body. These may come out in tears or words, and therapists are trained to listen and be supportive.

BENEFITS

Rolfing is believed to increase mobility, release musculo-skeletal pain and correct postural imbalances.

Craniosacral therapy

BACKGROUND

Craniosacral therapy was developed in the United States by John E. Upledger in the 1970s. It is a gentle hands-on treatment that is used to evaluate and enhance the craniosacral system to activate the body's natural healing mechanisms.

The craniosacral system is comprised of membranes and fluid, which surround and protect the brain and spinal cord. This therapy believes that restrictions or imbalances in the physiology of this system will negatively affect the functioning of the rest of the body.

Craniosacral therapy involves the application of very light pressure applied through the hands to the cranium, sacrum and any other appropriate part of the body to treat areas of imbalance.

TECHNIQUE

A treatment will last from 30 minutes to one hour. The therapist will listen to the recipient's body and use gentle palpation techniques at various points in the body to evaluate the craniosacral system and release any imbalances or tension, thereby encouraging the body to heal itself. Treatments are given with the recipient fully clothed.

BENEFITS

Craniosacral therapy is used for treating headaches, hormonal issues, fatigue and insomnia.

Reiki

BACKGROUND

Reiki comes from the Japanese words "rei" meaning universal and "ki", the word for energy, which has been discussed in the shiatsu and acupressure therapies. Reiki was introduced and developed in Japan by Mikao Usui; it is a gentle, non-intrusive method of hands-on healing.

Reiki is based on the theory of universal energy. This energy radiates in and around the body, but can become blocked through physical or emotional trauma, which may result in ill health. Reiki aims to re-channel, rebalance and replenish an individual's universal energy. If emotional or physical blocks are removed, the recipient can return to an optimal sense of wellbeing.

TECHNIQUE

A treatment can last up to one hour. It will be given on a massage couch or the floor with the recipient fully clothed. No oils are used. The therapist will scan the recipient's body, searching for energy blocks, by holding their hands a few inches above the body. They continue to hold their hands on or above the body at a series of positions, usually the energy centres (chakras), drawing the recipient's energy through their hands. The hands will be held in this position until the universal energy is released and starts to flow to the required areas.

BENEFITS

Reiki is advocated for clearing the mind, releasing stress and emotional blocks and reducing related pain.

Associations/ organizations

These associations and organizations will provide information on accredited courses and therapists.

BRITISH ASSOCIATIONS

International Federation of Reflexologists	e	ifr44@aol.com
	w	www.reflexology-ifr.com
Aromatherapy Regulations	e	info@aromatherapy-regulation.org.uk
	w	www.aromatherapy-regulation.org.uk
International Federation of Aromatherapists	e	office@ifaroma.org
	w	www.ifaroma.org
British Complementary Therapies Association (BCMA)	e	info@bcma.co.uk
	w	www.bcma.co.uk
The Shiatsu Society	e	admin@shiatsu.org
	w	www.shiatsu.org
The Ayurvedic Company of Great Britain	e	
	w	www.ayurvedagb.com
The British Massage Therapy Council	e	info@bmtc.co.uk
	w	www.bmtc.co.uk
The British Reflexology Association	e	bra@britreflex.co.uk
	w	www.britreflex.co.uk
The Sports Massage Association	e	info&thesma.org
	w	www.sportsmassageassociation.org
Manual Lymphatic Drainage UK	e	admin@mlduk.org.uk
	w	www.mlduk.org.uk
International Association of Infant Massage	e	mail@iaim.org.uk
	w	www.iaim.@org.uk
European College of Bowen Studies (ECBS)	e	info@thebowentechnique.com
	w	www.thebowentechnique.com

Bowen Therapists' **European Register (BTER)**	e info@bter.org w www.bter.org
The Reiki Association	e co-ordinator@reikiassociation.org.uk w www.reikiassociation.org.uk
The Rolfing Association	e info@rolfing.org w www.rolfing.org
Polarity Therapy Association	e info@ukpta.org.uk w www.ukpta.org.uk
Craniosacral Therapy **Association**	e office@craniosacral.co.uk w www.craniosacral.co.uk

AMERICAN ASSOCATIONS

American Organization for **Bodywork Therapies of Asia**	e secretary@aobta-md.org w www.aobta-md.org
Polarity Therapy Association	e hq@polaritytherapy.org w www.polaritytherapy.org
Acupressure Institute **of America**	e info@acupressure.com w www.acupressure.com
National Ayurvdic Medical **Association**	e info@ayurveda-nama.org w www.ayurveda-nama.org
IMA Group, International **Massage Association,** **Inc.**	e info@imagroup.com w www.imagroup.com
ABMP, Associated **Bodyworker & Massage** **Professionals, Inc.**	e expectmore@abmp.com w www.abmp.com
AMTA, American Massage **Therapy Association,** **Inc.**	e info@amtamassage.org w www.amtamassage.org
CMTA, Clinical Massage **Therapy Association,** **Inc.**	w www.clinicalmassage.com
NYSSMMT, New York State **Society of Medical Massage** **Therapists**	e jan2hoff@aol.com w www.nysmassage.org

American Association of Oriental Medicine	e	AAOM1@aol.com
	w	www.aaom.org
American Craniosacral Therapy Association	e	acsta@acsta.com
	w	www.acsta.com
AMMA, American Medical Massage Association, Inc.	e	rdeperio@americanmedicalmassage.com
	w	www.americanmedicalmassage.com
American Organization for Bodywork Therapies of Asia	e	www.aobta.org
	w	aobta@prodigy.net
Bowen Therapy Academy of Australia-North American Registry	e	usabowen@aol.com
	w	www.bowtech.com
FSMTA, Florida State Massage Therapy Association	e	info@fsmta.org
	w	www.fsmta.org
Hawaiian Lomilomi Association	e	lomidoc@lomilomi.org
	w	www.lomilomi.org
International Association for Holistic Aromatherapy	e	info@naha.org
	w	www.naha.org
International Association of Infant Massage	e	iaim4us@aol.com
	w	www.iaim-us.com
International Council of Reflexologists	e	quantum@ns.net
International Thai Therapists Association	e	itta@megsinet.net
	w	www.thaimassage.com
North America Vodder Association of Lymphatic Therapy	e	wellnessbp@earthlink.net
	w	www.navalt.com
Reflexology Association of America	w	www.reflexology-USA.org
Reiki Alliance	w	reikialliance@compuserve.com
Rolf Institute of Structural Integration	e	Rolfinst@rolf.org
	w	www.rolf.org
Rosen Method Professional Association	e	info@rosenmethod.org
	w	www.rosenmethod.org

(e e:mail address | w web address)

Index